LANDSCAPES OF CARE

Landscapes of Care
Comparative Perspectives on Family Caregiving

ANDREW POWER
National University of Ireland Galway, Ireland

ASHGATE

Published by
Ashgate Publishing Limited
Wey Court East
Union Road
Farnham
Surrey, GU9 7PT
England

Ashgate Publishing Company
Suite 420
101 Cherry Street
Burlington
VT 05401–4405
USA

www.ashgate.com

British Library Cataloguing in Publication Data
Power, Andrew.
Landscapes of care : comparative perspectives on family caregiving.
1. People with mental disabilities--Care--England.
2. People with mental disabilities--Care--Ireland.
3. People with mental disabilities--Care--United States.
4. Caregivers--Government policy--England.
5. Caregivers--Government policy--Ireland.
6. Caregivers--Government policy--United States.
7. Caregivers--Services for--Cross-cultural studies.
I. Title
362.3'8-dc22

Library of Congress Cataloging-in-Publication Data
Power, Andrew.
Landscapes of care: comparative perspectives on family caregiving / by Andrew Power.
p. cm.
Includes bibliographical references and index.
ISBN 978-0-7546-7950-9 (hardback) -- ISBN 978-0-7546-9888-3 (ebk)
1. Public welfare--Great Britain. 2. Great Britain--Social policy. 3. Public welfare--United States. 4. United States--Social policy. 5. Public welfare--Ireland. 6. Ireland--Social policy. I. Title.
HV245.P663 2010
361--dc22

2010017366

ISBN 978 0 7546 7950 9 (hbk)
ISBN 978 0 7546 9888 3 (ebk)

Mixed Sources
Product group from well-managed forests and other controlled sources
www.fsc.org Cert no. SGS-COC-2482
© 1996 Forest Stewardship Council
FSC

Printed and bound in Great Britain by
TJ International Ltd, Padstow, Cornwall

Contents

List of Tables

Preface

The care of people with intellectual disabilities is provided through a variety of sources. Of all these sources, the informal sector – made up of family caregivers – is the largest. This book is concerned with the geographies of carer support and how institutional structures at national, regional and local levels interlock to provide systems of care support. The book raises pertinent questions around the role of government, civil society and service providers in family support.

At the national level, state and voluntary services are analysed in the US, England and Ireland by examining how caregivers are 'targeted' by the different models of welfare. A post-structuralist perspective is used to examine how carers and care recipients are socially constructed across space and place, and how care discourses have manifested themselves in the actual provision of care services. Interviews were carried out with statutory and voluntary carer support agencies on how policies are interpreted and implemented on the ground in each country.

To explore these issues in more depth, this book examines the case of Ireland in more detail. Ireland has a very distinct history of support across scale and possesses a unique blend of Catholic *conservative* 'family' policy and 'neo-liberal' statutory provision. This forms a particularly interesting case study in examining broader debates in welfare and redistributive justice.

This case study is informed by the narratives of family caregivers who are affected by existing policy. Particular attention is paid to the everyday geographies of care and experiences of support services by the families themselves. The caregivers' accounts illustrate both the social and spatial difficulties of navigating through a landscape of care characterised by insufficient and conflicting information on services, a lack of shared knowledge between service providers and limited available services, and how these problems shape the caregiving experience within the home.

Acknowledgements

I would like to thank Professor Rob Kitchin and Dr Ronan Foley for their help, advice, encouragement and direction during my time at NUI Maynooth. The fieldwork during my time there was funded by the National Institute for Regional and Spatial Analysis (NIRSA).

I would also like to thank Brigid Barron, May Gannon, Claire Douglas, Paddy O'Shea, Winifred Quin, Christine Milligan, Tony Gatrell and Susan Reinhard for their help in getting (and keeping) the fieldwork off the ground. A quick thanks also goes to Phil MacMenamin, Holly Platt, Katrina Roen and Sabrina Mazzoni for their hospitable welcome abroad.

There are many friends and colleagues in both the Department of Geography at NUI Maynooth and NIRSA who I cannot mention individually, but whose kindness and helpfulness never went unnoticed.

Finally, special thanks must go to my family and my partner Jenny for their support and patience throughout the writing of this book.

Chapter 1
Introduction

> There are only four kinds of people in the world – those who are currently caregivers, those who have been caregivers, those who will be caregivers, and those who will need caregivers.
>
> Rosalynn Carter (former First Lady) *Helping Yourself Help Others*

Since de-institutionalisation began in the 1970s in many Western jurisdictions, family caregiving has been affected by an orchestrated set of policies and measures aimed at reducing state involvement in welfare provision. Home care has arguably been a victim of larger neo-liberal processes in which economic, socio-cultural, and political problems are displaced into voluntary services and the family in order to restructure state responsibility and save public finances. Support provided by family and friends is the critical foundation of community care. In particular, caregiving for young adults with intellectual disabilities is in large part determined by the resources of individual families and the mix of community services available. Often a lack of support mechanisms for carers can lead to other considerable social and economic costs such as family breakdown and institutionalisation.

Over the last decade or so, the landscape of care support within capitalist welfare states has become more and more decentralised, with increasing reliance on the voluntary sector. This has occurred after years of political and ideological debate about the potential for voluntarism to resolve their fiscal problems (Salamon et al., 2003). Parallel to this, there has been a greater tendency to introduce increased competition, procurement and contractual management across these states, for managing the relationship between the different actors within the welfare sector. The *Compact* in the UK and the *Accord* in Canada are examples of new ways in contracting with the voluntary sector (Plowden, 2003; Creese, 2006). This has led to a significant debate in social policy and new public management literature which discusses the relative merits of increased contracting and governance by the state in the nonprofit sector. Central to this debate are the effects on family caregivers themselves. Both the type and extent of family care have been shaped by differing political and socio-cultural constructions of care and how these have been interpreted within a framework of rights and responsibilities. As the book shall explore, this framework and the precise form of neo-liberalism that states have adopted are historically and geographically specific.

In discussing welfare systems and support provision, it is clear that they are about much more than the organisation of services or benefits; they are about how societies value different roles and responsibilities, and how major social divisions – such as class, gender, disability and indeed family carers – are conceptualised.

From the classification of social membership and personal need to the management of resources, social welfare is embedded in a wide range of political, economic and cultural discourses (O'Brien and Penna, 1998). The discourse of care thus holds considerable implications for the socio-spatial arrangement of care. These discourses have undergone significant restructuring in the wake of neo-liberalism, and consequently so have the packages of care provided to family carers. In light of these changes and in the context of new social movements centred on 'identity politics', the way in which a State constructs the notion of rights and welfare has become a key indicator in assessing care provision. Examining the differences across countries illustrates the relative impacts of their historical, social, economic and cultural contexts on the landscapes of care for family caregivers. Here, care is largely interpreted within a relational framework that examines the linkages between care-giving expectations, the context in which it occurs and those charged with its delivery.

Intertwined with this broader welfare debate over how best to support care providers, recent discourses on care have included a more fundamental debate around the contested nature of care itself, from those in receipt of it. Given the long history of paternalistic forms of congregated care and enforced dependency of people with disabilities, particularly for those with intellectual disabilities, there has been much resistance to varying social notions of care. Terms such as service user or client have served to replicate this resistance. The person is often viewed as a dependent recipient of care, rather than an active citizen being in reciprocal and interdependent supporting relationships. Such thinking has arguably continued to undermine or negate individuals' capacity for autonomy and self-determination (Thomas, 2007). This view continues to inform debates on care and independence. Hence, despite the shift to family care, the term 'care' is one that remains synonymous with dependency in disability studies (Oliver, 1996; Oliver and Barnes, 1998). Indeed, Twigg and Atkin (1994) go so far as to suggest that while informal (family) carers are by and large seen as part of the solution, they may also be part of the problem.

The complexity of understanding family care then, is obscured by the ways in which family 'informal' carers have become the subjects of debate themselves within health and social care policy in recent years. Twigg and Atkin (1994), for example, noted how family carers could (and were) being classified as service-users, resources, and co-workers. As a result, the intricacy of care relationships between family carers and other groups, has led to complex policy intersections, which in turn has had a substantial impact on the people involved and vice versa. Notable areas of work have therefore focused on the implications for who cares (Twigg and Atkin, 1994; Milligan and Power, 2009); as well as multiple definitions of care (Watson et al., 2004; Morris, 1993).

In the context of these debates, this book examines the discourses of care and the resultant landscape of caregiving policy for families caring for their young adult children with intellectual disabilities in three different jurisdictions; the U.S., England and Ireland. The comparative analysis unpacks these central debates regarding how care is viewed by the state and demonstrates the intricate interplay of historical, social, cultural and political factors in shaping such care policy. It shows that any attempt to 'read' the landscape of care cannot be undertaken without an understanding of the particular context within which it is situated. While there are some commonalities across the three jurisdictions, how care policy is manifest in each country is rather different.

In order to explore the impacts of these debates on family caregivers themselves, the book examines the local scale within Ireland in more depth. Ireland serves as a particularly interesting case study of what can happen to a care system when the state operates a decentralised 'relaxed-control' approach. Given its unique social history, particularly in terms of the influence of the Roman Catholic Church and state subsidiarity,[1] Ireland offers a distinctive perspective in unpacking these broader welfare debates, as well as examining the experiences of family members *within* the context of such contested notions of care. This book thus examines in more depth the social and spatial implications of its particular model on family caregiving on the ground. It provides a timely analysis of home care for families of people with intellectual disabilities in Ireland in comparison to England and the US.

The use of the term 'Landscapes of Care' in the title represents an attempt at presenting a critical study of the informal care sector and the *spatial* experience of care beyond a surface identification of spatial patterns. It draws on concepts in human and cultural geography which have a broader understanding of landscape as a humanistic and culturally constituted phenomenon that extends beyond a purely physical environment. The term in some ways builds upon Gleeson and Kearns' (2001) original concept, 'moral landscapes of care', in which they critically look at the moral geographies associated with re-locating care in the community. In their paper, they question the moral binary of presenting institutions as inhumane, and community care as nurturing and emancipatory. Rather, they advocate a critical perspective which goes beyond formulaic ideals of community care to try and identify a landscape which has a sincere and inclusive ethic of care. Similarly, rather than solely focusing on the physical caregiving infrastructure on the landscape, analysis is extended to examine how and why care ideology is structured and experienced as it is. At the comparative scale, this means examining the ideologies and discourses which underlie care support. At the local Irish scale, this means uncovering the lived experiences of those who deliver care, thereby placing them 'in' the landscape. Since community care is as much about private lives as it is about public policy, this book is thus centrally concerned with the way in which caregiving is experienced by those who live *within* a landscape of intersecting community care policies.

At the same time, the concept 'landscapes of care' echoes many of the themes emerging from the therapeutic landscapes literature, in particular the everyday milieu of caregiving in which a carer lives and the emotional ties between the

1 Subsidiarity became a guiding principle in Ireland's welfare policy, meaning the state did not become involved in social affairs, leaving the family and parish to develop local support arrangements.

individual and their 'place' (see Williams, 2002). On the one hand, 'landscapes of care' resonates with Gesler's (1992) original conception of therapeutic landscapes, articulated as 'settings or situations that encompass physical, psychological and social environments that are associated with healing [and wellbeing]'. The home for many carers and adults with intellectual disabilities can represent a haven from public scorn and awkwardness. However, on the other hand it is important to recognise that the familiar sites of the home and the 'in-between' social spaces in which care takes place are often simultaneously places of contestation, isolation and hurt. The therapeutic landscapes concept is thus better understood in this context as a dynamic and evolving process, in which the carer has to continually manage circumstances to help 'maintain' a therapeutic landscape of care.

Given the limited academic research on geographies of caregiving for young adults with intellectual disabilities and the broader comparative analysis of caring in geography more generally this book works towards two ends. Firstly, to develop a critical study of home care and to construct a cross-cultural comparison through charting the ideologies, provision and experiences of home caring in different countries. Secondly, to expand theoretical understanding in relation to the support provision and experiences of home care. This is achieved through incorporating the perspectives of post-structuralist theory to focus on the discourses of citizenship, social justice and care, in order to construct a moral geography of care.

Carers for Adults with Intellectual Disability

This book takes as its focus families caring for young adults aged 18 and above with intellectual disabilities. When an individual turns 18 years of age, there is often a significant transition from second-level education into adult services, and a different set of structures and benefits provided by the state. In general this is typified by means-tested assistance, day care services, and occupational and life-skills training. The progression into adulthood is one of the most significant transitions experienced by individuals and their families and a lot of planning and mentoring is required to set up sustainable and individually tailored supports for the person. This process is compounded by the young adult's capacity to make decisions, and the level of advocacy required in planning for future supports. As a result, this transition into adulthood often represents a significantly more stressful time for people with intellectual disabilities and their families. Leaving education for teenagers with learning difficulties may only serve to highlight differences from intellectually-able peers. It appears that the education system (whether mainstream or segregated), offers a secure environment that many families find it difficult to envisage their child ever having to leave. Most parents of young adults with intellectual disabilities worry therefore about their child's move into adulthood and are apprehensive about the uncertainty of the future (Redmond, 1996).

Intellectual disability[2] is a problematic and complex concept that is difficult to define. Generally, an individual with an intellectual disability has a greater than average difficulty in learning, there are difficulties with everyday life skills; and the condition is present from childhood. People often require alternate training methods and speech therapy in order to reach their full academic potential. However, the meaning and interpretation of intellectual disability are negotiable and vary across time and place. For instance, people with Down's syndrome can be highly independent, yet at the same time can be particularly vulnerable to dependency creation (Swain et al. 2003). They do not necessarily have a general learning disability; rather, they have a characteristic learning profile with specific strengths and weaknesses. There are factors that facilitate learning which can be used to offset factors that inhibit learning. While definitions of intellectual disabilities may provide some insight into the disability itself, it is important that these definitions do not overly label the person and that generalised assumptions are not made.

The role of caregiving for people with intellectual disabilities is thus a complex area, particularly given its contested history. 'Good' care can depend on the policy commitment to provide and design the most appropriate services, the level of funding made available, and the attitude of society in general towards those who have an intellectual disability. Good care also depends on how appropriate the caregiving relationship is, in relation to the needs and preferences of the individual. Moreover, it is important that such forms of care are not paternalistic, overbearing or restrictive.

Scales of Study

As Townsend (1995) has argued, welfare policy can no longer limit itself only to the national arena but must address the connections between the local and the global. Any narrative of health and social care restructuring must take into account the relationships between actors operating at various spatial scales (Milligan, 2000a). Addressing such connections also necessitates an encounter with political, economic and cultural forces. Given that carer support services are structured differently in each country, the book provides a comparative analysis of how services developed over time across three different jurisdictions (the US, England and Ireland) and the extent to which the services meet carer demand on the ground. While recent research is increasingly recognising the uneven geography of welfare, many of these descriptions have been static snapshots in time rather than dynamic, which makes it difficult to determine how policy developed over time (Powell and Boyne, 2001).

2 The term 'intellectual disability' was chosen as it is a generic and universal descriptor used across many jurisdictions. 'Learning disability' is more typically used in the UK.

The book is structured in three related parts, and the content makes a logical progression from the macro to micro scales:

- Part I examines the different concepts of welfare, citizenship, and rights and responsibilities related to care.
- The comparative analyses in Part II explore how different jurisdictions apply these notions in constructing their landscape of care. In addition, each chapter illustrates the models of citizenship and social justice from which the family carers (and their associations) draw their political strategies. In other words, the book seeks to examine the ways in which hegemonic discourses of welfare and care are being challenged by carers and those they care for, and to document alternative care strategies being pursued. This provides a context for considering the merits and limitations of how home care is institutionally and ideologically framed and in particular how various discourses (e.g. political ideologies, conceptions of citizenship and social justice) create and reproduce care support provision.
- Finally, Part III offers a more detailed case-study of whether institutional structures in Ireland interlock at regional and local levels to provide an effective system of care support. The analysis evaluates critically how carer support is spatially structured, the services provided, and how they target carers. An important component of this is an investigation into the experiences of carers themselves and how the care services offered shape their lives. Issues regarding carers in the community are held in focus with broader issues such as the contested history and notion of care, individual rights of the care recipient, citizenship rights, and the role of welfare.

A Note on Methods of Analysis

In order to examine the 'place' of caregiving within broader debates of welfare, the book aims to move beyond reductionist typologies of each country towards a deeper examination of their historical, cultural and political contexts. Therefore, in order to develop the international comparative part of the book, the methodological framework was based on a detailed examination of literature followed by site-visits to each country. The site visits provided a means to investigate the broader social factors such as different conceptions of disability, family responsibility, and role of community in each country.

Stage One

To move beyond the typologies and to provide a detailed examination of literature, a wide range of material needed to be consulted, across a range of disciplines, as well as from public, voluntary, and academic sources. Furthermore, a historical perspective was needed to trace how these discourses developed and changed over time, and so a detailed archival search was undertaken of policy and legal documents, organisation mission statements, media stories and book publications. Government and voluntary body websites were also consulted to gather data on welfare benefits, payments and entitlements. This was an ongoing process and continued throughout the later stages. This was supplemented by examining peer-reviewed journal articles and books in the field. The research throughout all the comparative chapters is heavily based on the policy and academic literature consulted.

Stage Two

The purpose of the site-visits was twofold: to facilitate getting to the hard-to-find 'grey' literature (including studies on health, welfare, disability, and caregiver policy) and to meet key academics and carer organisations to learn their thoughts on local community care practices. Because of the differing definitions and practices of carer support in each country, initial contact was made with the research staff at host universities, and from there, prospective interviewees were formed with key participants in the field.

For the English case-study, it was decided to base the research at the Institute of Health Research, Lancaster University, as a result of the presence of key researchers in the area of disability and care. Four weeks of fieldwork were undertaken – two weeks in May and two weeks in June 2003. Meetings were held with researchers at the Institute, drawn from the fields of social work, politics, and of community-care work, for the purposes of attaining a more detailed insight of English carer policy. Meetings then took place with local caregiver agencies during the June phase of the trip.

For the US case-study, the research was based at the Center for State Health Policy at Rutgers University, New Jersey. The institute hosted a visit in October 2003. Again, initial meetings took place with academic staff at the institute to gain local insight with US health and community care policy. This was followed up by meetings with local community organisations, as well as some national advocacy agencies in Washington D.C. and New York.

Unfortunately, it was not possible to interview individual carers during the site-visits due to time and cost constraints, as well as having to go through separate ethical approval for each jurisdiction. The body of literature consulted thus forms the major part of the chapter analysis at the national comparative scale. Although the meetings and interviews with academics and organisations were key to shedding light on carer policy, the discussion throughout the English and US chapters is mainly guided by the literature. This process was repeated one final time in order to develop the comparative chapter with Ireland. A detailed literature review of academic and policy reports was undertaken, followed by meetings with national advocacy organisations and the relevant government ministry.

Stage Three

The final part of the book largely portrays the experience of carers at a local level, within the Irish context. It offers a more detailed account of the implications of Ireland's particular and unique context. Therefore, in order to gain a deeper perspective than the broader comparative welfare analysis, a detailed inventory of care support services was undertaken, and was followed up by interviews with national carer organisations, regional health authorities, service providers, as well as family carers between Autumn 2003 and Spring 2004. The inventory documented all forms of support services offered to home carers and the qualifications needed to avail of such services.

In order to move beyond this 'quantification' of the landscape of care support, interviews were then conducted with the five national carer organisations. There were two separate themes addressed in the interviews. Firstly, they tried to tease out the agencies' views on carers' issues and concerns. Secondly, they intended to probe organisations on their views of the family care policy climate, including issues related to their own relationship with Health Service Executive Areas (formerly Health Boards), service gaps, funding and resource issues, organisational aims and objectives, and changing relationships within and between organisations and the State.

In terms of the statutory agencies, interviews were conducted with key informants from the Health Authorities within three study areas; the Northern Area Health Board, the South Western Area Health Board (both within the Eastern Regional Health Authority), the Western Health Board, and the Midland Health Board. The interview questions focused on what services were provided, how decisions were made on the particular service provision, and what were the main service gaps which they were aware of.

In terms of the service providers interviewed, a small sample of four intellectual disability service provider agencies was selected that the families were using within the two regions; the South Western Area Health Board (SWAHB) and the north of the Northern Area Health Board (NAHB) (two in each). These were the main intellectual disability service providers in each area, and provided a range of supports including a day centre, independent living training, occupational training, friendship and social development support, respite, and so on. These agencies were non-profit grass-roots organisations that did not provide residential support like some of the larger predominantly Church-based institutional services.

Finally, the book also attempts to explore the narratives of family carers themselves. Twenty-five interviews were conducted with carers in the Co. Kildare and north County Dublin. These were chosen to represent carers in a suburban area (north county Dublin) (n=7) and in a semi-rural commuter area (Kildare) (n=18). Table 1.1 outlines the main demographic details of the interview sample. Twenty-two of the carers were women, however, alongside the three male carers interviewed, some female carers spoke of shared caregiving between themselves and their male partners. The most important aspect of the sampling was to identify

Table 1.1 Profile of Family Carers Interviewed

No.	Gender	Age Group of Carer	Age of Recipient	Disability of young adult	Region
1	Female	50–60	18–25	Down Syndrome	Co. Kildare
2	Female	40–50	18–25	Down Syndrome	Co. Kildare
3	Female	40–50	18–25	Developmental	Co. Kildare
4	Female	50–60	18–25	Down Syndrome	Co. Kildare
5	Female	70–80	40–50	Down Syndrome	Co. Kildare
6	Female	40–50	18–25	Autism with learning difficulty	Co. Kildare
7	Female	40–50	18–25	Down Syndrome	Co. Kildare
8	Female	40–50	18–25	Down Syndrome	Co. Kildare
9	Female	40–50	18–25	Autism with learning difficulty	Co. Kildare
10	Female	70–80	40–50	Down Syndrome	Co. Kildare
11	Female	40–50	18–25	Autism with learning difficulty	Co. Kildare
12	Female	40–50	18–25	Down Syndrome	Co. Kildare
13	Female	40–50	18–25	Developmental	Co. Kildare
14	Female	40–50	18–25	Down Syndrome	Co. Kildare
15	Female	40–50	18–25	Down Syndrome	Co. Kildare
16	Female	40–50	18–25	Down Syndrome	Co. Kildare
17	Female	40–50	18–25	Autism with learning difficulty	Co. Kildare
18	Female	40–50	18–25	Down Syndrome	Co. Kildare
19	Female	40–50	18–25	Multiple disability	N. Co. Dublin
20	Female	60–70	18–25	Down Syndrome	N. Co. Dublin
21	Male	50–60	18–25	Down Syndrome	N. Co. Dublin
22	Male	60–70	18–25	Down Syndrome	N. Co. Dublin
23	Female	60–70	40–50	Developmental	N. Co. Dublin
24	Male	40–50	18–25	Down Syndrome	N. Co. Dublin
25	Female	40–50	18–25	Down Syndrome	N. Co. Dublin

those caring for adults with intellectual disabilities, thus the majority of caregivers were caring for people within the 18–25 group who had gone through the child-to-adult transition relatively recently. It was made clear that the respondents had the right to expect that any information they provided would be treated in confidence. Because of the sensitive nature of the book, the anonymity of those who participated in the interviews has been protected.

The main issue explored in these interviews was how the broader debates of care and the landscape of supports shaped the daily experiences of carers. As part of this, the relationships in which informal care took place were examined, not just as caring relationships, but as social relationships. This was achieved by investigating caring activities and their meanings for the participants through locating them in their social setting. Thus the result should offer a picture of the *social context* which helps to account for the kind of giving and receiving of support which takes place (or fails to take place).

Book Structure

The book is divided into nine chapters, across three interconnected parts. In Part I, following the introduction, Chapter 2 examines the concept of family care itself. It traces the changes in how carers have been defined within community care practices and presents the patterns of carer support that have emerged in today's context. It examines important and topical issues of gender and disability critiques of care, before exploring how a spatial perspective can be useful in unpacking many issues in caregiving research, such as the real environments in which caring takes place.

Chapter 3 develops the core conceptual framework of the book regarding the discouses of care within contemporary welfare, and the implications they have on family carers. It explores the key concepts around landscapes of care, specifically family care, welfare and citizenship as they apply to families of adults with intellectual disabilities, and broad critiques and theorisation around these. The rights ascertained from citizenship and the entitlements from welfare are key to understanding the scope of recognition of carers from a state. The chapter therefore details the rise of social rights and the construction of the 'welfare state' as it exists today. To engage with this question further, the last section outlines the development of a theoretical perspective through which one can make sense of contemporary welfare systems and provision. The analysis of national policy for carers draws upon the strategies of post-structuralism to enable both criticism and re-imagination of traditional political-economy approaches generally used in cross-country comparisons of welfare. An anti-essentialist notion of carers is developed to allow room to uncover how the identity of carers in each country has been constructed over time, and how this has fed into different institutional practices in community care. This sets the context for a deeper analysis of the statutory and voluntary sector in Ireland and abroad.

In Part II, Chapters 4, 5 and 6 examine the legislative and welfare systems of England, the US, and Ireland respectively. As policy makers around the world consider ways to reduce the tensions between work and family responsibilities, and the question of appropriate roles of governments, employers, workers, and the voluntary sector, the book examines the experiences within these three nations, in how they have grappled with these debates. Rather than giving a typology of each country, each chapter attempts to examine the historical, social, cultural, and economic contexts in which care support is delivered. Each chapter aims to trace the way in which contemporary welfare and disability policies have created institutions and modes of practice, which have had a direct bearing on the circumstances of carers' lives.

Part III of the book, in order to advance the narrative beyond national comparative contexts, begins a more thorough examination of the broader care debates within a case study of Ireland. Chapter 7 deals with the regional allocation of care in Ireland and examines the government's role in service provision. It focuses on the workings of the contemporary Irish State and how their welfare policies filter down through both regional and local level. In light of this analysis, Chapter 8 draws exclusively from interviews with carers themselves in order to examine their everyday social and spatial experiences and unpacks the physical, emotional and psychological effects of being within such a landscape of care. Concepts of space and place are shown to be helpful in understanding issues and experiences of caregiving such as how carers deal with promoting independence, yet struggle with overprotection, in different spatial settings.

Finally, the conclusions in Chapter 9 offer an assessment of how the discourses of care in each country have led to fundamentally different directions in community care policy. It argues for a broader conceptualisation of care support and promotes the idea of a wider caringscape closely allied with community development, rather than advocating for more narrowly defined carer respite.

PART I
Concepts of Care

Chapter 2
Family Care

Discourses and Debates of Care

Western ideology currently holds that the care for people with disabilities is best provided in a home environment. Government since the 1970s have been intent on moving away from institutional forms of care to care within, and arguably *by*, the community (Coppock and Hopton, 2000). The tipping of the balance towards increased caregiver responsibilities and the rolling back of the state in many neo-liberal countries over the last decade has led to a backlash from carer groups against policy makers who neglect the extensive work carried out by families, and an upsurge in interest from social commentators and feminist scholars(discussed below).

The ideal of care in the community in which those with an intellectual disability could live a full, inclusive life nurtured by those around them is still fraught with many challenges. While the care of people with disabilities comes from a variety of sources: the state, the private market, volunteers and family and friends, of all these sources, the informal sector of the family remains the largest and most fundamental. Community care is often a synonym for family care, often without the promised support and resources necessary for the system to function properly (Barnes, 1997).

Services had their origins in first blaming then neglecting families (Noll and Trent, 2004). Families were later 'rediscovered' by policy makers who found that they were the kernel of support in the community. As a result, over the last two decades a vocabulary of care has become incorporated into welfare policy. In constructing the concept of family carer (or 'caregiver' in North America), there has been much working and reworking of the term as research and policy interest in caregiving has gathered pace. It has developed a more specific and more complex meaning than just referring to the daily roles and relationships that are constructed through the practice of looking after people. Caregiving is heterogeneous and dynamic by nature. As a result, different and sometimes conflicting notions of care exist.

Abrams (1978) in his study of care networks, is credited with having introduced the distinction between informal and formal care, where informal care is defined as unpaid care based on personal relationships, and formal care as paid care that is provided within a framework of bureaucratic rules and regulations. In other words, informal care is that which is thought to exist 'naturally' in the community, provided voluntarily by spouses, siblings, children, and close and distant relatives (Lane et al., 2000). Formal carers, such as attendant care professionals, generally work for an agency and are paid to go into people's homes to help out with some of the everyday duties which the care recipient requires, thus indirectly relieving the informal carer. Formal care is usually sporadic in nature as a result of practical constraints such as workload, the scale of service, and the availability of finance. Even if the care given by professionals in the community is informal in nature – such as providing emotional support – it is not defined as informal care.

Because of its kinship-base, the relationships between carer and care recipient constitute a 'sector' rather than a 'system' of care. Unlike other sources of health care – the private market, the state and the voluntary sector – caring in the informal sector does not integrate the carer into an organisational structure of carers. According to Graham (1999), despite being sometimes called the 'informal system', 'community care', or 'army of carers', the informal sector is characterised by literally thousands of separate carer-care recipient relationships where individual carers work on their own. The language of care and its different meanings is thus important, as it can have different effects on the way carers are represented and targeted by policy. The following sections within this chapter unpack the varying discourses and debates which have emerged in relation to the concept of caregiving.

With regard to the actual terms used in this book, 'carer' is used to denote the individuals involved in informal caregiving, whilst the term 'informal care' is used to describe the resource or 'service' that they provide within the social care network.[1] The current favouring of the term *carer* has probably confused many families in practice, particularly for those who have cared for a long time, when less than forty years before, the term 'carer' was barely in the English language (Bytheway and Johnson, 2008). Many still identify themselves as 'a mother caring for her disabled son or daughter', for example, without fully comprehending the extent to which their duties transgress most 'normal' experiences of managing home duties. In some ways, it represents a 'concretising' of an identity and is often shaped by policy makers' and professionals' views of the relationships involved. Despite its heterogeneous and dynamic nature, advocacy groups often encourage people to identify themselves as 'carers' – in recognition that caregiving is a job that transcends familial responsibility. A survey by the National Family Caregiving Association (2000) in the United States for example, found that self-identification does make a positive difference in the attitudes and actions of family caregivers, in that it makes them realise they are not like other family members who would look after a 'normal' child. It is therefore an important goal to be pursued, according to the Association.

Faced with the dilemma of wanting to make positive claims for certain groups while simultaneously acknowledging individualism, often a process of 'strategic essentialism' (coined by Chakravorty Spiva, 1988) is involved in which one can speak in rather simplified forms of group identity for the purposes of struggle while debating within the group the finer shades of difference. However, while

1 Family carers often do not like being called 'informal carers', hence the choice of the more generic term 'carer'.

representative groups like above often hold onto broad definitions of care, the methods, purposes and results of this concretising need to be examined. A critical stance towards the 'taken for granted' construction of the identity which engages with the multiple and contested different forms of care needs to be developed.

One of the foremost oversimplifications of family care involves the concept of the 'family' itself. Despite the differences in sizes, compositions, and rates of divorce, separation and single-parenthood, the conventional nuclear family model is still presumed. Indeed, rates of divorce and single-parenthood are often put forward as representing the demise of the family (Jones, 2002). However, it must be asked did a golden era of conservative families and strong kin relations exist? In reality, a closer look at families throughout the twentieth century reveals a different picture. Ireland for example, had one of the highest rates of single unmarried people in Europe in the early part of the last century, yet the role of the family was ceremoniously idealised in the Constitution (McLaughlin, 1994). Policy makers in particular have created highly normative values of family functioning (see Commission on the Family, 1998). Importantly these ideological assumptions can have profound effects on carers, whose families do not 'live up' to the homogenous units often portrayed. This raises debates over obligation, duty, love and solidarity – and who provides care. Phillips (2009) identifies that in reality, ambivalence is likely to be found increasingly in intergenerational relations as complexity and diversity characterise family relations and lifestyles. However, claims that the family is 'disintegrating' should perhaps be treated with caution as empirical studies (Williams, 2004) appear to capture the variability of how people experience family life, rather than its complete collapse.

Another area of debate in caregiving relates to the 'paid' and 'unpaid' dichotomy (Daly and Lewis, 2000). Although informal care is to a large extent unpaid care, much has been argued about this unwaged/waged dichotomy. It has been claimed that the introduction of state payments for carers are an example of how the boundaries between these two forms of care are being removed (Ungerson, 1995). However, informal care is not based on a formal contract of employment or a code of professional ethics like most positions. In addition, informal carers very often have to depend on piecemeal welfare benefits as a result of the need to forfeit employment in the workforce. Hence they are normally supported by limited and limiting government financial support and mainly third sector service provision. Therefore they reduce significantly the potential burden of cost incurred by the State. In addition there are many additional costs such as the direct expenditure on medication, food, laundry, and arranging disability transport. Therefore their enormous contribution in terms of time and effort often goes relatively unnoticed and unpaid.

Another debate which has emerged regarding the various definitions and expectations of care is the way in which the care relationship is framed with the *recipient* of that care. Often notions of care can cast the recipients as dependent, passive and intert relative to caregivers. This can sometimes lead to contestation by certain sections of the population. Indeed, the disability movement has been very resistant to notions of care being prioritised, arguing that the carer agenda often places disabled people as being dependent with negative, powerless implications for them as individuals and as 'burdens' on the family (see Oliver, 1990, Shakespeare, 2000). The word 'care' has been described as 'ideological dynamite' (Oliver and Barnes, 1998: 8). They argue that, '[c]onstructing the category carer and developing policies in respect of this group has neither enabled disabled people to become independent nor freed other family members from their "caring" duties' (Oliver and Barnes, 1998: 8).

This has led to much debate over the role of carers in the lives of persons with disabilities. The term care, as the later comparative chapters shall examine, has for a long time been synonymous with traditional, paternalistic, and often custodial forms of support. During the heyday of asylums in the 1800s, governments used the idea of 'moral treatment' as a basis for providing care for persons considered 'mental defectives' in segregated environments (Finnane, 1981). However, as early as the late 1800s, calls for their closure were being made. For example, in 1894, the superintendent of the Richmond asylum in Ireland warned his colleagues that asylums were not conducive to recovery, nor even to a tolerable existence for many of their inmates; 'It would be better for many patients to be outside, boarded out with sympathetic families' (Finnane, 1981: 185). Despite these warnings, the system of institutionalisation continued to dominate the Victorian landscape of care across the Western world.

The legacies of these institutions have arguably lived on, in particular in the working culture and mindsets of people involved in the persons' care. According to the European Commission (2009), institutions should no longer be defined primarily by their size but above all by features of 'institutional culture' (depersonalisation, rigidity of routine, block treatment, social distance, paternalism). Size is merely an indicator – the larger the setting, the fewer the chances are to guarantee individualised, needs-tailored services as well as participation and inclusion in the community. Despite the change in the site of care, the medicalisation and bio-reductionism of individuals with disabilities is thought to have remained in the newer infrastructure of community care.

Similarly, Oliver (1996) warns that the change to care in the community potentially still creates dependency – it has simply been repackaged within a new frame of practice. With the long history of paternalistic and professional intervention, those involved in caring are held responsible for creating and exacerbating dependency by denying people with disabilities the means by which to govern their own lives. The earlier paradigm of the person being helpless is argued to still live on in the practice of many medical and social care professionals, who assume paternalistic positions of power and control over the lives of disabled people, thus undermining or negating a person's capacity for autonomy and self-determination (Thomas, 2007). Here, such a dominant medical view within care practices is likened to the concept of 'disablism', which refers to the social beliefs and actions that oppress, exclude and disadvantage people with impairments (Abberley, 1987).

This view continues to inform debates on care and independence. Hence, despite the shift to community-based care, the term 'care' is one that still evokes deep feelings of distrust. Moreover, it has been argued that 'family care' is not exempt from dependency creation. According to Morris (1993), it neither guarantees greater independence nor autonomy for disabled people. Moreover, Twigg and Atkin (1994) go so far as to suggest that while family carers are by and large seen as part of the solution, they may also be part of the problem. Similarly, authors such as Swain (2003) argue that people with intellectual disabilities may be particularly over controlled by their parents and carers and denied opportunities for experimentation and choice. At the same time, a person with an intellectual disability may find it difficult to initiate change and parents may be reluctant to do so because of upheaval, risk and threat to existing sources of support.

This perspective is contrasted by much of the earlier carer literature, particularly from the women's perspective, which emphasised the burden on women from the roles and obligations involved. This burden has been described in numerous ways, including feelings of burnout, depression, isolation, sadness, fear, anxiety, grief, and loneliness (Murphy et al., 2007). Within this literature, caregivers have reported higher levels of depression and psychological distress, a more negative affect, and higher use of psychotropic drugs than people in the general population (Cuellar and Butts, 1999: 24). Clearly then, the women's and disabled people's movements hold very different, if not contradictory, positions and priorities with respect to care (Milligan and Power, 2009). To examine this further, the gender perspective is explored in more detail below.

Gender Issues of Care

One of the key issues touched on above is that of gender. Caring is predominantly tied up with women's identity, particularly for women who are socialised into servicing or nurturing roles. As a result, the most comprehensive research that has developed on 'informal care' has arisen in feminist literature on the family. The feminist critique of community care emerged in the early 1980s and has continued throughout the 1990s and 2000s (see Finch and Groves, 1983; Ungerson, 1990; 1995; Graham, 1999; Cranford, et al., 2005). Its earlier literature challenged the traditional sociology of the family and pointed to the way in which kinship obligations are 'gendered'. The origins of studies on informal care lay in the continuation and extension of feminist debates concerning childcare, the role of women's unpaid labour and the significance of the family in public policy (Twigg and Atkin, 1994). Informal care was therefore defined as part of the kinship obligations of close female relatives.

The image of family support as the domain of women, especially in relation to the kind of assistance which entails practical, personal and domestic tasks, comes through strongly in the earlier tradition of British kinship studies (Finch and Mason, 1999). These studies often resorted to women's altruism as an explanation for this. Many writers (Rose, 1993; Holloway, 1999) who have worked in feminist geographies have critiqued this assumption. Whatever the source of the motivation, altruism can hardly explain why people provide care beyond levels that is good for their own health and well-being. Land and Rose (1985) describe the normative social pressure of this sort as 'compulsory altruism'.

Finch and Mason (1999) found that both male and female responses to who should carry out domestic responsibilities is more ambiguous than one might expect. However, these gendered patterns usually only emerge or become clarified when people are pushed to make a choice. In other words when families find themselves with little choice to take on the caregiving of a relative, there is often not as much open discussion and choice as normal. In practice 'shared care' between family members is uncommon, often other relatives withdraw once a main carer has been identified (Finch and Mason, 1999). Therefore there are two levels of gender role recognition: In the first instance, when in a non-crisis situation, there can be an amenable 'equal shares' solution. In the second instance when in a more critical situation, there tends to be a more definite gendered choice. For instance when faced with an immediate family dilemma, such as discovering that a child has a disability, the woman more often takes over the role of personal care. There is a difference then between normative statements and reported experience. Finch and Mason (1999) points out that people do not carry around with them stable sets of values and meanings, but construct them, when they have to, out of the various materials available. There is often little choice for the women involved when it comes to making a decision as to whether or not to care.

A woman having once taken on the role of carer, may find herself caring for one dependent relative after another and is therefore caught in what Rimmer (1983) calls a 'caring cycle'; that because she has cared for one relative, she should carry on this personal role for another and perhaps another. This is seen to lie in women's responsibilities for the care of able-bodied partners and children. Women find themselves engaged in the care of other kin because they are engaged in the care of their immediate family. This has also been referred to as 'women in the middle' (Brody, 1981) to characterise women who, after relinquishing the demands of child care, are called on to provide care for their ageing parents or parents-in-law. Twigg and Atkin (1994) argue that it is women rather than men who are most likely to find themselves engaged in caring for the family across the life-cycle, working as principal carers through this 'cycle of caring' (Twigg and Atkin, 1994).

Gender issues of caregiving also continue to be debated in the formal care literature. For instance, Cranford et al. (2005) illustrate the difficulties faced by low-paid women in care-attendant jobs in the shadows of the direct payment movement in Canada. This movement has been largely led by people with physical disabilities, centred on giving individuals with disabilities more choice in their support arrangements. One of the knock-on effects however, has been a driving down of the cost of care, resulting in lower pay and less security for care workers, and resistance to a unionised care workforce. Ultimately, this has affected the large rate of single mothers and female migrants involved in this work.

While these studies have conceptualised the different gender roles, few studies have explicitly looked at male carers. This is despite the fact that the percentage of male carers in early research studies ranged from 23 per cent to 41 per cent of the samples (Arber and Gilbert, 1989). Moreover, in the 1985 UK General Household Survey, there was an unexpectedly high proportion of male carers, which Arber and Ginn (1990) credited as 'spousal care', where older husbands were caring for ill wives. As a result Bytheway and Johnson (2008) calls for a disaggregation of carers to recognise the multiple different carer relations, including the 'forgotten male carer'. This clearly does not make redundant the feminist critique of informal caring, but has meant that it must take account of the increasingly complex issues of family obligations and characteristics of care. Similarly, Phillips (2007) argues that even with mens increasing involvement in care, particularly in working class families, gender stereotypes still exist.

Behind these trends found in the literature, there exist many gender assumptions which are built into political debates concerning the nature of family relationships and the responsibilities associated with them. Analysis of the concept of care needs to expose the gender ideology that informs the policy agenda. Yet at the same time, given the rates and roles of male caregiving, we cannot either be gender neutral in our analysis of care or use a gendered lens to see the concept as a 'women's issue' (Phillips, 2007). As touched on earlier, the type and extent of care which takes place within the family is likely to be at least partially determined by the nature of the family in the society under study. Factors such as the type of family organisation and the way in which the family as an institution is perceived by that society need to be considered as well as the extent of familial contacts and the degree of affectivity within individual families and so on. Care is perhaps best defined then through its complexity, given that it involves all aspects of life, and is subject to differing social, political, ethical and cultural interpretations (Phillips, 2007). These varying interpretations can lead to different material responses in the form of supports. Often 'care' within policy is constructed as charitable non-work provided by philanthropic women (National Council for the Elderly, 1994). This highlights the importance of not only examining carer policy but also to try and trace the origins of how the discourses used in the welfare state engender this distinction.

Geographies of Disability and Care

Another essential aspect in understanding care is the multiple ways in which geography can affect the lives of the carer and care recipient. In particular, the location of care of people with disabilities affects everyday care practices. The geography of disability literature has explored the myriad ways in which disabled people have been and continue to be spatially segregated by care arrangements. This segregation in turn shapes family interactions and caregiving relationships.

Geographic enquiry into the 'care' of persons with disabilities developed initially from critiques of the spatial segregation of asylum care. The work of Philo

(1987) drew attention to the way people with mental illness were removed from society and placed in asylums. This became a burgeoning field of research within health geography, as reflected by the two special editions on the asylum within *Health & Place* (1997, 2000).

In terms of post-asylum geographies, Pinch (1985) and Dear and Wolch (1987) first examined the social exclusion and service dependency experienced by many disabled people, particularly in urban cities. Since these earlier studies, the social model of disability, defined as a rejection of the dominant biomedical understanding of disability as a condition that has to be cured (see Oliver, 1990) has informed much of the geographical literature. Morris (1991) and Imrie (1996) looked at how the spatial layout of the built environment has been constructed in a way that complements and reinforces their marginalisation. According to Kitchin (1998) space is organised and planned for the benefit of non-disabled people. State policy, building regulations, architectural and planning practice and budgetary concerns combined with individual social interactions all have a role in constructing these environments. This has been referred to as the 'design apartheid' where the city is designed as if all people are the same (non-disabled) (Imrie 1996). Importantly in this literature, disability was recast as a socially constructed entity, rather than a biological certainty (Hall and Kearns, 2001).

In addition to the geographical literature on the built environment, geographers found that the experience of inaccessibility and exclusion is shaped equally, and perhaps more tellingly, by the attitudinal environment (Hawkesworth, 2001). This arose largely from the post-asylum geographic research on those with mental illness. According to Morris (1991):

> It is not only physical limitations that restrict [people with disabilities] to our homes and those whom we know. It is the knowledge that each entry into the public world will be dominated by stares, by condescension, by pity and by hostility (1991: 25).

As well as the exclusion of those with physical disabilities, Parr (1995) found comparable socio-spatial relations amongst individuals with mental health problems. She found that the attitudinal environment makes it difficult for the person to carve out a wider personal and spatial life.

Sibley (2001: 363) argues that the integrity of a person is threatened when the spatial partition of a boundary is transgressed. In other words it was not by accident that people with disabilities were separated from society in the past. Wilton (1997) draws on psychoanalytic theory to examine how people's own sense of identity is to some extent dependent upon the maintenance of surrounding social and spatial order. The supposed threat is minimised when the social distance is 'sustained and complemented by spatial separation' (Wilton, 1997: 461). Dear et al. (1997) examined how the production of difference is characterised as necessarily a social and a spatial process which allows the self to be *partitioned* from the 'Other'. Entangled with this concern is the question of how identities are constituted, acted upon, and become 'fixed' or maintained (Dyck, 1998: 104–5). Hence, the processes that create boundaries that exclude people with disabilities are social and at the same time necessarily spatial. The process of situating self in space, often involves imposing a literal boundary between self and Other (Sibley, 1995). Therefore there is a link between access to space and identity. The immediate presence of difference and the transgression of established boundaries run counter to the well-being of individual identity because they challenge the territorial position of the self (Wilton, 1997).

This focus on the social representation and cultural construction of disability and its spatial implications led some geographers (Butler and Bowlby, 1997; Hall, 2000) to comment on the failure to acknowledge the real pain and exhaustion caused by a person's impairment. This failure is largely a result of the dominant focus on the social model of disability. In response, Hall (2000) states that as well as facing the disabling processes from society, the actual bodily impairment is also a very real concern. Geographers must take the body seriously in the analysis of health and impairment. He argues that recent geography literature has understood 'the body' mainly as representation. He maintains that a blurring of the usual polarities of biology and society is important. As Dorn and Laws (1994: 107) point out, we need 'an understanding of the body in both its material and representational forms'. A notable exception to this omission has been the work of Isabel Dyck (1995) who examined the changing everyday geographies of women with multiple sclerosis. She found that the majority of women were found to experience shrinking social and geographical worlds due to physical impairment as well as exclusionary space.

While this work on the geographies of physical disabilities and mental illness has certainly brought the debates in how people with disabilities have been treated forward, and undoubtedly resonates with many of the experiences of people with intellectual disabilities, a specific geography focusing on this group has only emerged quite recently. This literature has engaged predominantly with the community based care locations and structures, which have been set up to place people in the community. Wolpert's work (1976) for example, examined the lives of people with intellectual disabilities in group homes, co-operative housing, residence with parents and some independent housing. Similarly, Radford and Phillips (1985) and Metzel (2004) in their analysis of community care housing invariably found that the large, spatially isolated asylum had been replaced by the apparent freedom of a life in the community which very often is life in an 'asylum without walls' (Dear and Wolch, 1987). With group homes, there was much antagonism and ignorance in communities at neighbourhood level. Many people still exhibited nervousness, fear, and basic ignorance to people with disabilities (Wilton et al. 1997).

More recently, a paper by Hall and Kearns (2001) entitled 'Making space for the "intellectual" in geographies of disability' kickstarted a special issue on the subject in the same journal (*Health & Place*, 2005). Its publication was timely, as despite community care being accepted as the strategic vision of most government's disability policy, evidence of isolation, lack of jobs, and impoverishment had increased within the intellectual disability population (Emerson, 2007). Geographers have since attempted to provide more nuanced readings of the complex geography of intellectual disability. Much of this work has attempted to destabilise various assumptions regarding the 'most suitable' place of care. The traditional binaries between spaces of institutionalisation/deinstitutionalisation, isolation/integration and success/failure have been challenged. Hall's (2005) work in particular has scrutinised the entangled geographies of social exclusion/inclusion for people with intellectual disabilities. Drawing on group interviews in Scotland, he develops a nuanced account of the lives of individuals, exploring their experiences of exclusion and seeming 'inclusion', and also the alternative spaces and networks of inclusion that they had developed. His paper argues that we must be critical of the spaces of incorporation and not assume a place of incorporation is the best choice for a person with an intellectual disability. This is particularly evident in the public sphere, where people with intellectual disabilities often face a mix of patronisation, fear, an unwillingness to understand 'non-standard' forms of communication, and a strong sense of difference. Thus while people with intellectual disabilities continue to prove over and again that they are capable of far more independence than many had expected, and policy makers, researchers and 'advocates' gain a vision of greater changes that are possible, at the same time, there is an honest recognition within this literature that people with intellectual disabilities can still be susceptible to isolation and discomfort in 'inclusionary' spaces.

While this literature has certainly considered in various ways, the 'care' of persons with disabilities, the ways in which family care relationships are involved have been more often than not neglected. An explicit geographical analysis on family caregiving of adults with intellectual disabilities continues to be a significant gap within the literature (although see Ryan's 2008 paper on caring in public space for an exception). Much of the geographies of care has focused on home care given to the elderly (Milligan, 2009; Twigg, 2000; Wiles, 2003) and the chronically-ill (Thomas and Morris, 2002). This geographical work has in many ways placed geographers at the cutting edge of conceptualising care. The two main strands within this work have been the examination of home care service provision (Fyffe and Milligan, 2003; Williams, 1996) and the changing nature of the home space (Milligan, 2000; Williams, 2002; Wiles, 2003).

In terms of the first strand, geographers have looked at how home care programmes are set up and how policies have contributed to geographical inequalities that exist in home care services throughout a region. For example, Williams (1996) examined the importance of the economic, social and political factors in the evolution of long-term care policy in Ontario. Such an approach, she posits, recognises that both economics and politics contribute to the power relations that are particularly important in the differential distribution of power and resources between groups. Also within this strand has been an examination of the geographical perspectives on voluntarism and social welfare (Fyfe and Milligan, 2003). Inherent in this work is an acknowledgement of the mixed model of welfare provision for carers and the consequences on the availability, accessibility and quality of services. Addressing the challenges of providing home care programs in rural settings has also been a concern of geographers, where there are limitations in healthcare access (Cuellar and Butts, 1999).

In terms of the second strand (the changing home space), the spatial domain of care has tended to be characterised by the terms *public* and *private* (Twigg, 2000). These are useful terms because they enable geographers to identify how the private nature of the home can change with significant care demands. The household as the site of caregiving is problematic and awkward because it is the setting that traditionally has been considered a refuge from work and public interference (Rosenberg, 1987). In contrast to institutional care settings, family care is embedded in intimate, affective relationships that have histories and futures. Hence, home care is delivered in a complex interactional context which is characterised by tension as well as solicitude and warmth (Atkin, 1992). The work by Wiles (2003), for example, examines the profound spatial and social impact of providing informal care to an elderly family member on their everyday home space. She focuses on the themes of mobility and routine and the inter-relationships of scale to show how caregiving can constrain their daily geographies. Again, disrupting sites of care is an important point in analysing this relationship. As a result of the increasing intercession by the state, market and voluntary sectors in the home, the home site can become one where there is a blurring of private and public. As Milligan argues, domestic space can be seen to have merged with public services to become a site of caring (2000b). She argues that in situations where there is no option of alternative sites of caring such as day-care, the restructuring of care into the home may be more aptly described as 'an institutionalisation of the carer's private space' (p. 55). The home space is also seen to become a site of work for the carer, thus adding to a growing complexity of the home/work space. Therefore it is suggested that the provision of formal and informal care within the home space is creating a new site of caring in which both private (informal) and public (formal) must merge.

Williams (2002) employs the concept of *therapeutic landscapes* as a framework in examining the place identity and the meaning of home space. The therapeutic landscapes concept, as identified earlier, has been articulated as a setting or situation that encompasses physical, psychological and social environments that are associated with healing and wellbeing (Gesler, 1992). While there is much greater understanding of the impact of caregiving on family carers, Williams (2002) acknowledges that little is known about how care in the home affects the physical and social environments for those who live there. While the home can operate as a therapeutic environment for the ill and the dying, it is not known if this exists for young adults with intellectual disabilities or the family caregivers involved in their lives. Donovan and Williams (2007) in their analysis of palliative caregiving, illustrate the ways that caregiving significantly alters family caregivers' experience of home but, with adequate support (physical, emotional and financial), the potential for the home to be therapeutic indeed exists. Understanding these complex spatial experiences of care suggests a potential to grapple in a new and productive way with the idea of therapeutic landscapes by relocating some of that discussion into the every day worlds of unpaid carers of adults with intellectual disabilities and those adults themselves along with the political-institutional arrangements that support them. This would be a useful conceptual contribution to geographical debates on care as well as broader discussions on care.

As mentioned above, one notable contribution to this literature has been Ryan's (2008) paper which examined the effects on family caregivers of adults with intellectual disabilities in public space. Her illustration of the reactions to disability in public life, such as stares, pity and negative comments, and parent's consequential coping strategies, serves to demonstrate the importance of geography in discussions of caregiving for people with intellectual disabilities such as deciding on places to go and how to act in these places. As Hall and Kearns (2001) argue, people with intellectual impairment have generally been characterised as leading 'inconspicuous lives' (p. 240), which may have contributed to inhibiting public awareness. For example there is often a greater sense of spatial exclusion through segregated 'special schools', 'special' transport, sheltered work, and social contact (Baron et al., 1998). This spatial exclusion helps to produce and re-produce the self-identity of intellectually disabled people as dependent and vulnerable.

This book builds on this disability and caregiver research by focusing on the socio-spatial experiences of carers of young adults with intellectual disabilities. More specifically, it examines how their experiences can be intrinsically different to those caring for people with physical disabilities and mental illness and at different stages in the lifecycle. As a result of the time-investment involved by carers in the monitoring of behaviour and routine, often the care of adults with intellectual disabilities remains a relatively invisible and geographically small world. In addition, in response to Wolch and Philo's (2000) call, the focus on the materiality of everyday life 'must go beyond the local, immediate experience of the individual and be set within, and connected to, the context of economic and socio-spatial reform and transformation' (cited in Hall and Kearns, 2001: 244). To meet this end, a comparison of how different states have represented and targeted carers of adults with intellectual disabilities serves to address the relative absence of this form of care in the geographies of disability and care.

Chapter 3
Welfare and Care

With the advent of community care, the State has left itself in a paradoxical situation. On the one hand, it has promoted care in the community, and for the independent living of the person with a disability. On the other hand, it must provide the financial resources and the community infrastructure to reach this aim; the spending for which goes against many western, neo-liberal ideas of government. This chapter examines this paradox and the concept of neo-liberal governance, with respect to its perceived role in supporting family care. The chapter raises important questions around the role of government in family support. It concludes by identifying the theoretical framework for examining the comparative case-study chapters.

Welfare refers both to the health, happiness, and fortunes of a person or group and to the actions or procedures designed to promote the basic and material well-being of people in need.[1] These procedures can include transfer payments to those unable to work and the guaranteed provision of certain essential elements of a 'decent' standard of living, like health care, and education. The organisation of welfare in capitalist societies is complex and multi-faceted. People derive their welfare from a range of institutions and sites, so that the organisation of welfare involves labour markets, families, voluntary and state agencies, charities, and so on (O'Brien and Penna, 1998). However with the rise of liberalism and citizenship rights, came an incremental separation of public and private spheres, thus changing the discourses regarding the 'right place' for women as carers (Isin and Wood, 1999). This chapter examines the historical evolution of welfare itself as a concept and how this change came about. It also highlights some of the different models of welfare provision and how carers themselves fit in, or 'are targeted' by these different models of welfare. Key to this is the idea of citizenship, and a country's understanding of it. As part of exploring welfare, the chapter also focuses on the geographical issues of welfare, such as allocation, access, and utility.

Liberalism and the Rise of Citizenship Rights

The term 'citizenship' and its related language of 'rights' have become very common in popular discourses within mainstream society. Often carer organisations and sympathetic media features make the call for better carers' rights. However, the particulars of both terms have often become over simplified. Generally, T.H. Marshall's work (1950) is cited as the most significant contribution to the literature

1 According to the *Oxford English Dictionary* 2010.

on rights. His early work argued that a modern society involves the enjoyment of three basic types of right – civil, political, and social – each of which developed in a rough historical sequence. Although there was much overlap, in essence, civil rights first started in England in the 17th and 18th centuries, political rights in the 19th century and social rights in the 20th century. In the late 20th century, there was also an emergence of 'cultural rights' across the world as a consequence of identity struggles based on gender, race, ethnicity, and sexuality. These are dealt with towards the end of the chapter. The growth of rights in general were dictated by specific historical events that took place rather than a logical progression (Isin and Wood, 1999). Much of the way they were cultivated was based on the social struggles that surrounded the development of liberalism and its modern counterpart, neo-liberalism.

The start of civil rights can be traced back to the British *Bill of Rights* (1689), which composed the first constitutional monarchy in the world by stipulating that the execution of laws by regal authority, without consent of Parliament, was deemed illegal. However, despite the *Bill of Rights*, no constitution really protected British subjects from political abuses. The King had the full power of creating Lords; he therefore had an influence over legislation (Biscay, 1999). In response, John Locke was credited with drawing up individualistic rights to life, liberty, and estate, of which the political state could not interfere. In *Two Treatises of Government* (1690) he had two purposes in view: to refute the doctrine of the Divine and absolute right of the Monarch and to establish a theory which would reconcile the liberty of the citizen with political order (*Encylopaedia of Philosophy*, 2001). The response was to insist that government may act only in the interests of the freedom of the individual; that government had no wider role in the organisation and regulation of civil life; that the only legitimate basis of government was to maintain a legal framework in which individuals could follow their life's goals without undue interference from others. It was seen to be a move away from such governing powers where rule was derived from the greatness of the Monarchy, to a system of procedural (legal) rules. As long as these rules are applied impartially to all, then the state is 'moral' (O'Brien and Penna, 1998: 19). This set a precedent for the rest of the western world.

The philosophy of liberalism began to take shape from this time and the idea of minimal state based on governing by procedural rules was formulated most clearly by Adam Smith who drew on many of the philosophical and economic theories of this period. Although the main tenets of his work, *An Inquiry into the Nature And Causes of the Wealth of Nations* (1776), argued that self-interest can lead to social harmony – through competition and the mechanism of market demand – he believed the market to be self-regulating in that consumers' individual wants work as an 'invisible hand' to regulate supply and demand. This leads to a stabilisation where, although society would always remain stratified, he believed the level of riches enjoyed by all of its members would rise through the accumulation of capital. The contemporary use of liberalism by the New Right has arguably lost much of the subtlety of Adam Smith's writing in favour of an unabashed celebration of the excesses of the free market (Hutton, 1995, cited in Hubbard et al., 2002: 177). Furthermore, in Book Four of this work: *Of Systems of Political Economy*, he clearly sees a role for government and legislator, which has been largely ignored by neo-liberal governments:

> Political economy, considered as a branch of the science of a statesman or legislator, proposes two distinct objects: first, to provide a plentiful revenue or subsistence for the people, or more properly to enable them to provide such a revenue or subsistence for themselves; and secondly, to supply the state or commonwealth with a revenue sufficient for the public services. It proposes to enrich both the people and the sovereign. (Smith, 1776)

As long as the state was impartial, free of the distorting interference of organised monopolies or politically motivated social bodies, the wealth of nations was assured. He was well aware that it would not lead to an equalisation of individual wealth but to 'a stable, well-ordered and contented society where all persons enjoy sufficient wealth to leave behind the earlier feudal and early industrial world' (Smith, 1776).

The start of civil rights proper can be traced back to legislation concerning the freedom of the individual, such as the Factory Laws enacted from 1840 onwards which provided the individual with the ability to participate in the development of the industrial capitalist model (Biscay, 1999). The aim was to uphold individual freedom enabling citizens to take part in the decisions that create or re-create the contours of a society, like freedom of speech, thought, and faith. It also includes the right to own property, the right to justice, and equality in front of the law (Richardson, 1998).

In conjunction with the Factory Laws, political rights developed from the 19th century onwards. Under popular pressure, the *1832 Reform Act* in England abolished unrepresentative seats in Parliament in order to increase representation. It was seen however as an extension to those who, using their civil rights, had made economic gains and purchased property. They guaranteed the right to vote, the freedom of participation in the political process, and to join political organisations (Richardson, 1998). Even after the *1832 Reform Act*, the numbers of voters represented no more than one fifth of the adult male population. It was only in the second part of the 19th century that the extension of voting opened Parliament to the working class (Biscay, 1999). It gave industrialists and manufacturers a larger say in government than they ever had before.

One of the major effects of this reform period was legislation to detach political economy from domestic authority including the familial and the private sector. This greatly added to the gendered division between public and private, and the disenfranchisement and exclusion of women. Thus arguably the construction of women as carers in the home was copperfastened at this time. It effectively meant a system of rule in which 'state' and 'household' would be formally distinct. Even at this early stage, there was a manipulation of Enlightenment philosophy and a distorted theory of welfare. For example, women and the poor were denied many civil and political rights, based on the assumption that they were 'unable to be full citizens' (Isin and Wood, 1999: 27). The free-marketeers drew on controversial concepts of social inequality, for example, that the poor and uneducated did not know how to behave politically in a free way, which had distinguished Enlightenment origins (O'Brien and Penna, 1998). Thus both civil and political rights were in fact necessary to the development of capitalism and its class system by giving each adult male the right to engage as an independent agent in economic struggle (Isin and Wood, 1999).

The gap between philosophical liberalist thought and the political economy from this time widened. Early liberal government effectively tried to remove from the state any responsibility for provision against poverty or disability except in the most extreme cases of destitution. Another progressive liberalist thinker, Condorcet (1795), was strongly democratic and advocated universal equality of rights such as education and the reduction of poverty. Yet again however, his ideas were manipulated for the political liberal 'project'; those not educated in the 'correct' way did not fit collective life, or those who were impoverished were to be excluded because they were ignorant of enlightened action (O'Brien and Penna, 1998). The reform of the Poor Law at this time instituted the system of workhouses in which persons who could not support themselves were to be incarcerated.

With this liberalist thought, old forms of relief were believed to undermine the incentive to work. The basic tenets of capitalism – or the market – is that it recognises and rewards inequalities, and depends on them to provide the motive force that makes it work. This process was given free rein, as with 'laissez-faire' policy between 1845 and 1848 in England and Ireland. Thousands died of malnutrition or disease in Ireland and enormous numbers of English fled to the slums of bigger cities of Liverpool, Manchester and London. Liberals had their eyes on the prize of enlightened well-being *in the future* when the benefits of following natural economic laws would secure those goals (O'Brien and Penna, 1998: 24). In geographical terms, many Marxists have argued that the increase of wealth in one area necessarily creates poverty in another area, thus producing a recurrent inequality between both regions (Harvey, 1982). If left unchecked, the inequality between regions can become insurmountable. Liberalists argued that inequality (as distinct from *poverty*) is an essential structural feature. Some traditional liberalists even went as far as advocating the necessity of poverty, as expressed by Patrick Colquhoun when he described poverty as 'a most necessary and indispensable ingredient in society', because 'it is the source of wealth' (quoted in Marshall, 1977: 18).

The second wave of liberalism took place in the second half of the nineteenth century. Liberals such as John Stuart Mill in *Principles of Political Economy* (1848) viewed state action in social and civil life as a necessary evil; government would follow similar economic ideas but let welfare pick up the casualties. Even though this wave of liberalism contradicted some of the building blocks of early liberal political economy, it was accepted that such complex societies could no longer be left unregulated. In welfare, they promoted *formal* equality before the law for all (tax-payers) but did not promote equality in a *substantive* sense. They believed political rights accompanied personal and social enlightenment, a sort of moral paternalism. Around the same time, Charles Darwin published *The Origin of Species* (in 1859). Whilst Darwin's theories referred to *biological* evolution, they were themselves quickly 'adapted' by liberals, such as Herbert Spencer (1857), to apply to *social* evolution for such a cause. Many therefore considered liberalism a system which regards poverty as a weeder-out of the unfit, or as the inevitable and perpetual deposit of personal failures in the competitive struggle.

A third wave of liberal philosophy came about with some renowned economists and politicians in the 1920s and 1930s, such as Keynes, who renounced the basic principles of classical liberalism while still claiming the name 'liberal' in contrast with overtly collectivist economists (Huber and Stephens, 2001). The thesis as put forward by Keynes was that free market economics failed to deliver social stability, but at the same time recognised the major strength of enabling the pursuit of individual innovation, creativity and profit in a framework that did not predetermine what choices could be made. After the Great Depression of the 1930s in the US, the problem was how to ensure that the uncertainties of the economic system neither condemned capitalism, led to prolonged stagnation nor led to rampant social divisions (O'Brien and Penna, 1998: 35). The belief in the evolutionary benefits of poverty such as those from earlier traditional liberalists, were largely abandoned.

Social Rights and Welfare Protection

It was only in this third wave of liberal philosophy in the 20th century, with the rise of trade unionism and the right to bargain collectively, that social rights emerged. The development of state-supported elementary education in the 1800s was a decisive step towards the establishment of social rights in the following century. Also military involvement played a role as there was an extension in rights and privileges in exchange for service (Isin and Wood, 1999). It was to be much later that carers were established as a category under which social rights could be acceded. The main aim of social rights in Britain was the reduction of class conflict. This gave rise to egalitarian principles, the rise of real incomes which closed the gap between classes, and the development of mass production; which had the knock-on effect of the widespread incorporation of the working class in mass consumption. This had a profound effect on class inequality. The state no longer merely attempted to 'abate the obvious nuisance of destitution in the lowest ranks of society. It assumed the responsibility of modifying the whole pattern of social inequality' (Marshall, 1977).

Welfare came about then in response to these ideals of social rights. Indeed, Marshall's theoretical work largely examined the relationship between citizenship and the development of the welfare state. It was seen as an antidote to the impulsive nature of the market and the inequities of a society based on the principle of individualism, which refers to the process by which welfare entitlements are determined on the basis of individual status, rather than a familial one (Pfaller et al., 1991).

This realm of social rights is where much uncertainty has arisen in discourses regarding the role of the state. In theory, Marshall's notion of social rights responds to the social inequalities that threaten civil and political citizenship. He defines the social element as: 'the whole range from the right to a modicum of welfare and security to the right to share in the full social heritage and to live the life of a civilised being according to the standards prevailing in the society' (Marshall, 1950: 10–11). Unlike political and civil rights, which aided the development of capitalism and its class system, social rights have been argued to be in conflict with capitalism. According to Marshall (1950), 'those who were cautiously extending [rights] down the social scale probably did not realise quite how great the danger was [towards capitalism]' (cited in Isin and Wood, 1999: 29). Social rights generally include economic security, access to education, entitlement to work, and health services. According to Peillon (2001), through the enjoyment of a range of social rights, all differences including social, economic and cultural, are theoretically transcended. In that sense, citizenship upholds universal values, which do not erase differences, but works as a framework that endorses such differences and allows them to coexist harmoniously (p. 19). In other words, the aim is not *sameness*, one approach to all persons irrespective of their personal circumstances. Instead, it should aim towards implementing different approaches to achieve the sameness of *outcome*.

Although this is in essence the principle of the modern Western welfare state, in practice, as the next three chapters will examine, the welfare states of the US, England and Ireland developed very differently to each other as the ultimate responsibility of the state differed due to the local political, cultural and social context. Overall though, social rights, in contrast to civil and political rights, are largely viewed as political programmes, and are therefore depicted as involving high levels of state expenditure and intervention. It therefore becomes an issue of whom the state values more. Hence, the structure of the welfare system, and the range of rights are much more than the organisation of services or benefits; they are about how mainstream society views the responsibility and social role of its members. In this way, such rights are argued by many not to be 'rights' at all, but instead are akin to party manifestos (Drewett, 1999: 116–17).

In more recent times, *corporatist* structures have emerged within the welfare state leading to agreements between social partners (government, labour, and business) in the 'national interest'. The implication of this is that disabled people's access to social and health services, on the basis of rights, is much less developed than anti-discrimination measures and broader civil rights matters. In other words, the range of social rights which are supported very much depends on how society values and categorises the different divisions of people – such as class, gender, ethnicity or sexuality – as well as the cost. It does not cost much to 'recognise' the equality of some groups as they do not need support in the traditional sense. Marshall (1950) argues that social rights has made citizenship the architect of a new class inequality, as it can operate as an instrument of social stratification (cited in Isin and Wood, 1999).

More recently, the modern welfare state is under threat from a variety of fronts. Changing demographic patterns, declining public trust, interest group demands and growing international competition for capital and labour are presenting modern states with intense pressures (Deakin et al., 2004). Pfaller et al. (1991) posed the notion that the increase in international competition towards the end of the 20th century would lead to an even harsher challenge to the Western welfare states, and to the pursuit of non-economic objectives. Also structural forces within society such as institutional resilience show how past practices and policies all significantly affect current options in different ways. This is seen in the way the principle of *individualism* – the extent to which welfare can be tailored towards the individual – remains very limited or even deceptive in many countries. For example, the role of Church had a very important impact on the way the family was viewed by mainstream society in many European countries. This institutionalised traditional conservative-religious values in welfare policy such as familialism, which supported the male-breadwinner/female-carer model with cash transfers. The influence of religious social teachings remains a restraint on state provision of services, particularly those related to social care and family social reproduction. For instance, Ireland's welfare system still boasts its centre of attention to be the family unit (Department of Social Community and Family Affairs, 2001). According to Jones (2002), 'there was a powerful commitment to the ideological significance of the family as the care unit of society within the welfare state' (pp. 15–16).

This was mirrored in Britain and the US with reference to the number of women in the workplace after World War Two. In an effort to bolster traditional family forms, women were being encouraged out of the factories and back into the home. More recently, community care policy, seen as an evolution of state welfare strategies, puts very clear emphasis on the role of the family (Jones, 2002). The political ideology which gained popularity with the new rising white collar strata upheld the view that the responsibility of looking after the material needs of wife and children rests on the husband, while women assume responsibility for caring within the family (Esping-Andersen, 2000). This tied in strongly with the ideology that women are not perceived as autonomous individuals. Thus much like civil and political rights, there was a very deliberate separation of male/female, public/private in social rights. Caregiving in liberal thought is constructed as very much a private and female enterprise.

The fact remains that the needs of carers' is a recurring phenomenon in the western world, and neo-liberal governments take for granted the task of alleviating societies' problems jointly with welfare and capitalism. Generally, the welfare state as we know it today is a result of the interplay between social democratic and neo-liberal agendas. In recent years, economic globalisation and the economic policy guidelines promoted by liberal economists remains fashionable in the key centres of global development. However, as the following section shall examine, since the 1960s, a new form of identity politics and associated rights has emerged.

Cultural (Group) Rights

The history of liberalism and citizenship has until this point been considered purely in an evolutionary scheme and has exclusively focused on citizenship as social rights. However, the very concept of citizenship has since been called into question. The emergence of social movements and identity politics from the 1960s, based on ethnicity, gender, age, sexuality, disability and others have questioned the traditional universalist assumptions of redistributionist social policy, which extolled the civic virtues that created the basis for a moral community. Examples include the Black civil rights period and the women's movement in the 1960s and 1970s in the US. According to Marshall (1981), rights leaders were not asking for power over, or redistribution, but rather the power of recognition. In other words, they did not want to seek admission into American society as it was; they wanted a new American society that recognised all difference. Since then, in postmodern society the uni-dimensional nature of traditional social politics has been challenged by identity politics. The new disability movement, for example has posed major challenges to national collectivist discourse in a society which has traditionally screened out alternative perspectives. The universalism of the Welfare State is challenged by particularism arising out of the replacement of class-based social inequality by individual social movements, all concerned with their own recognition of their identity and attendant rights (Powell and Guerin, 1997: 45).

Group rights were first identified in Marshall's later work (1977), when he acknowledged a new call for 'rights of recognition'. This desire for recognition explains best the nature of group rights. The lack of freedom about which individuals or groups struggle, is usually related, as often as not, to the lack of proper recognition. The new welfare state has therefore had to come to grips with cultural or group rights, as well as the social rights it had granted, which traditionally took the form of universal access to health, education and so on. Debate surrounded the question of how much diversity could be accommodated within structures designed to foster unity.

As a result, citizenship is perhaps better understood as not purely a legal concept but also a sociological concept: It is not only conceived as a set of legal obligations and entitlements which individuals possess by virtue of their membership in a state but also conceived 'as the practices through which individuals and groups formulate and claim new rights or struggle to expand or maintain existing rights' (Isin and Wood, 1999: 4). In everyday life, being a citizen has recently been defined as the 'right to symbolic presence and visibility (vs. marginalisation); the right to dignifying representation (vs. stigmatisation); and the right to propagation of identity and maintenance of lifestyles (Pakulski, 1997: 80). The term group rights is closely linked to solidarity, fraternity, mutual understanding, and the need for association on equal terms (Isin and Wood, 1999). In other words, where the traditional aim of citizenship had been the dissolution of differences, there was a call by different segments in society to enforce the right to be different. Many groups that call for rights today, including carers' organisations, are not merely interested in abstract arguments about the common good; they are seeking legitimate recognition and citizenship rights.

It is worth noting that group rights initially existed in the medieval city, before the rise of liberalism and modernity, between the 9th and 19th centuries, in the form of guilds, cities, leagues, and communes (Gierke, 1990). The transformation occurred when modernity went from an inexhaustible combination of identities exercising group rights to only two sovereignties being recognised: the state and the individual (Gierke, 1990: 168–81). According to Isin and Wood (1999), modernity never solved the riddle of group rights. Since this period, the relationship between identity and citizenship has become essential to understanding cultural or group rights; in how individuals and groups identify themselves, and how citizenship grants rights to those identities. As group markers, the difference between citizenship and identity is that, while the former carries legal weight, the latter carries social and cultural weight. Citizenship can thus be thought of as a concept of status. Ultimately it allows or disallows civil, political and social rights (Isin and Wood, 1999). The modern state at the start of the 20th century exercised hegemony over these group multiplicities through suppressing them with a master national identity; in the interest of the 'national good' (Balibar, 1995).

This period of group rights' claims highlighted the shortcomings of traditional universalist aspirations of citizenship. Differentiated citizenship claims, or identity rights, according to Redden (2002), enrich the conceptual debate over social rights and citizenship. However for carers, the question becomes how to formulate a conception of citizenship and identity that enables the rights of carers. This debate is most acute when trying to make distinctions between those services which target directly the 'carer', and those services which target directly the 'core-recipient', which may also benefit the carer indirectly. Twigg (1992) refers to the former services as direct services, and to the latter as indirect services. However in many cases a distinction between direct and indirect is not always clear-cut. In terms of indirect services, it was found that improving the disabling environment and assisting the disabled person to participate in the ebb and flow of everyday life can indirectly be of great help to the family carer (Drake, 1999: 166). In terms of direct services, it has also been argued that helping carers can be very often one of the best ways of helping the people they are caring for (Holland, 2001).

Many problems exist with targeting carers however due to the complicated issue of citizenship. As Pakulski (1997) argues, the notion of what constitutes a 'good' citizen (recognition), and who is therefore entitled to rights (sanctioning), are the issues around which citizenship is contested. The notion of duties is important here, in which membership rights are twinned with responsibilities. The twinning of 'rights with responsibilities' is an issue that appears regularly in the literature on citizenship. We see for example that writings on sexuality have shown that it is the state that primarily defines which sexual activities are 'inappropriate' and uses constructions of morality to define the civil and welfare rights of its subjects based on their sexuality. This thinking is institutionalised in the law, and in tax and welfare systems (Kitchin and Lysaght, 2003). In these cases, the state and the legal system play a significant role in defining the citizen status of 'dissidents' who do not fit into normative roles. These roles are shaped by political rhetoric, religious doctrine, medical theory and the media.

It becomes clear however, from looking at other marginalised groups such as carers, that being allowed full citizen entitlements does not only entail being a 'good' citizen. Trying to be a 'good' citizen is often not rewarded when the state has conflicting ideals of what that behaviour should be. In the case of women, their 'natural' roles have become so embedded that they are not included in any measure of productivity, thus their role as a 'good' citizen goes largely unrewarded. It becomes apparent then that the notion of what constitutes a 'good' citizen does not only mean being 'good'. It means being 'good' at something which is laid down and rewarded by the state.

The Fabian ethic of duty – an understanding of citizenship based on rights being twinned with responsibilities – is therefore a lot more narrowly defined in reality. Given that legal rights and entitlements continue to be defined and anchored to nation-states, it is those who can contribute the most to the state who can expect the greater civil respect. In other words, those who pay more through consumer spending and tax offerings can expect greatest dignifying representation and symbolic presence. It therefore appears that citizen status can be bought in the guise of consumer status, something difficult for many carers given their economic position.

This situation leaves carers in a difficult position. Although they carry out demanding and arduous work in concurrence with the Fabian ethic of duty, their work goes largely unnoticed. Because their duty has historically been seen as nothing more than the regular maintenance of the home and family, the political and religious institutions accorded no extra symbolic or cultural status to such a duty. They therefore forfeit any extra entitlements which would seem appropriate to their work. Furthermore, the fact that they are not in a position to 'buy' their status as a citizen means they cannot avail of many of those entitlements offered to full citizens.

In combating this issue, one way of achieving emancipation for carers has been to try and give credence and symbolic capital to their social role. The method of *social role valorisation* has been employed by disability organisations to promote or 'give value' to their social role. Similarly carer organisations employ related techiques as a way of endorsing their duty as a viable and valuable mode of work. The importance of identity, both in how they perceive themselves, and how they are perceived by society and polity, is key to an approach for analysing carers' place in the world. Given that welfare and citizenship rights are given a privileged place in discussions about meeting carers' needs, the next section discusses how separate models of welfare have developed to reflect the local differences in understanding social roles and identities.

Models of Welfare

The modern welfare state is now in a very different position to that of Beveridge's post-war welfare effort. As the nature of citizenship rights have changed, welfare has had to structure arrangements to accommodate new and ever-changing social and cultural rights. An essential criteria in defining welfare states is the quality of these rights, the degree of social stratification and the relationship between state, market, voluntary and community sector, and family. Throughout history, differences in how these factors have been conceptualised have led to the composition of distinct welfare regimes across the world. These regimes are basic models which refer to the ways in which welfare production is allocated (see Esping-Andersen, 1999). The following definition is useful;

> A regime is understood as a particular constellation of social, political and economic arrangements which tend to nurture a particular welfare system, which in turn supports a particular pattern of stratification, and thus feeds back into its own stability. (George and Taylor-Gooby, 1996)

The concept of different welfare regimes has been discussed for a long time. Richard Titmuss (1974) provided one of the earlier attempts, making a distinction between 'three contrasting models or functions of social policy' – residual, handmaiden and institutionalist models – which have informed most latter typologies of western welfare provision arrangements. Under the residual model of welfare provision, social services are provided to people who are unable to help themselves. They form a safety net which catches individuals temporarily when the 'natural' channels of welfare (the private market and the family) break down. Under the handmaiden model of welfare provision, social needs are met on the basis of 'merit, work performance and productivity' (Titmuss, 1974). Under the institutionalist model, services are provided on a universal basis and social welfare as an integrated institution in society, 'providing universalist services outside the market on the principle of need' (Titmuss, 1974).

Similarly, Esping-Andersen's seminal work entitled *Worlds of Welfare* (1990) also classified models of welfare into three *regimes* based on similar types of structure: conservative-corporatist, social democratic, and liberal. In the first instance, social entitlements derive principally from *employment* (as in Germany). The core structural characteristics of this welfare state consist of occupationally based social insurance. In the second instance, social entitlements are derived more fundamentally from being a *member* of the country (as in the Nordic model). It is distinctively universalist in its policy approach. Social Democrats do not simply favour financing generous schemes of redistribution, they strive to promote social equality more generally through full employment policies and generous social services for all classes. Finally, under the Liberal welfare state, entitlements are based on *proven need* (as in the more targeted systems in North America). The state therefore has a residual duty to provide for those unable to provide for themselves, which in modern market society is determined through market earnings. The Liberal system is characterised by a disproportionate reliance on means-tested and private benefits and they are supposed to be sufficient just to cover bare subsistence needs. Liberals are anxious for welfare regimes not to create 'disincentives', discouraging people from paid labour. People are therefore primarily responsible for their own welfare.

Accompanying the State's welfare role is the voluntary and community pillar, made up of networks of third sector service providers, self-help groups, and charity and religious organisations. These organisations often provide essential services for the State or fill gaps in services neglected or underfunded by the State. Voluntary organisations have been defined as;

> self-governing associations of people who have joined together to take action for public benefit. They are not created by statute, or established for financial gain. They are founded on voluntary effort, but may employ paid staff and may have income from statutory sources. Some, [but] by no means all, are charities. They address a wide range of issues through direct service, advocacy, self-help and mutual aid, and campaigning (Taylor, 1992: 171).

While defined and conceived of as a sector, voluntary organisations are characterised by diversity in sources of funding, services, internal structure and autonomy (Clarke Cochrane, and Gewirtz 2001). Services offered can be seen to range from tangible provision such as domiciliary-based respite and personal care: visiting and befriending schemes; practical home support (e.g. meals provision, cleaning and home maintenance tasks, provision of practical aids); day-care and day-centres; transport schemes for elderly/disabled people; to non-tangible services such as support, advice, information and campaigning (Milligan and Fyffe, 2004). Voluntary organisations operating can also be differentiated by their size and organisational structure, i.e. those who are locally-based and independent of any hierarchical structure; those who are locally-based but affiliated to a national body; and those who are essentially 'satellite' organisations answerable to a national body.

In addition, there has been a new order of voluntary organisations which have arisen out of the emergence of cultural (group) rights' claims. They have been set up through pressure for bottom-up change as a result of a loss of confidence in the State. The range of critiques of welfare focusing on the particular experiences of different social groups has emerged from the so called 'new social movements', which include disability and the development of 'user movement' groups – the collective organisation of groups who use welfare services. The latter consist of self-advocacy groups for people with learning difficulties, for example. In some cases the new social movements and user movements overlap (Clarke, Cochrane, and Gewirtz, 2001). Civil society is therefore a contested terrain within which individual and collective actors compete to interpret needs and values as well as determine how social resources should be distributed (McGrath and Clutterbuck, 1998).

As the following chapters shall examine, throughout history, the contextual backgrounds of the relationships between state, market, voluntary and community sector, and family have led to the composition of distinct welfare and care regimes across the world. The aim of this book is to go further than labelling the case-studies as regimes and tease out the individual characteristics of the three jurisdictions examined. Esping-Andersen makes clear that there is no single pure case of the regimes he identifies. Scandinavian countries, for instance, are not free of liberal elements. Each particular welfare state will have elements of all three in its make-up, and some may have quite distinctive features. In order to move past this broad classification, it becomes necessary to carry out more detailed studies of individual states, both in order to go below the level of official statistics and explore the content of welfare policies, and to fill in some gaps, to understand why particular welfare states do not quite fit the various regimes. Geographers are uniquely placed to examine the unique social, cultural and political contexts of place in affecting the local arrangements of welfare.

Geographical Issues of Allocation

The geography of health and welfare provision is inevitably tied up with issues of resource allocation, priority-setting, or 'rationing' of services. Government constraints on health care expenditure mean that they cannot provide all the care a State might wish to and therefore decisions have to be made about the nature and range of services to provide. These are questions of a geographical, as well as an economic, political, and managerial nature, since such services will have to be provided some*where* (Gatrell, 2002, author's emphasis).

There is generally geographical disparity in the availability and provision of treatment and services (Joseph and Phillips, 1984). In most cases, political parties have developed a range of cost-control strategies as part of their ideology to bring credence to their political agendas and a way of rationing such services. Often, these involve control measures to be put in place to avert crisis away from them, as ambitious political agendas come into conflict with tight budgetary constraints. This enables them to present social programs to the electorate, while controlling the costs of such programs, through such methods as means-testing and restrictive definitions for eligibility. Current and forecasted demographic pressures in many Western countries have created strong incentives to examine strategies for controlling the costs of these programs that are targeted primarily or exclusively to the dependent portion of each State's population.

Kane's (1997) analysis of cost control in long-term care highlights how different nations have developed their own strategies for controlling social welfare expenditure. For example, many neo-liberal nations have some type of means-tested social assistance. What matters is the extent of restrictiveness of these tests and the generosity of benefits. Also, despite the universality of some countries' welfare provision, often the availability of care resources varies greatly between different parts of the country, such as in Scandinavian countries, for example, due to their long history of decentralisation (Byrkjeflot and Neby, 2008).

Looking across states, some common issues can be discerned. There are never enough resources to meet the demands for domestic social programs. The higher the fiscal impact of the proposed policy, the higher the impulse to narrow its scope. Some limitations and trade-offs are inevitable (Reinhard, 2001). When making decisions about the redistribution of limited resources, there are certain key criteria that can be adopted. Firstly, a government can aim to provide services that are *efficient.* This means the question of how to provide services that maximise outcomes while minimising cost. Secondly, a government can aim to provide services that are *effective*. In other words, are the treatments offered having real benefit, or are resources being wasted? Thirdly, a government can aim to provide services in an *equitable* way; are services being provided uniformly to the populations they are designed to serve? (Gatrell, 2002).

Equity in the provision of services must not be confused with equality however. Geographically, equality suggests that there should be an even distribution of services per head of population. But what matters much more is equality in relation to *need*, and this is what is understood by *equity* (Gatrell, 2002). When say, all poor citizens are provided with the same quantity and quality of medical care with approximately the same expenditures in time and distance, it is said there is *horizontal equity*. When both affluent and poor citizens are provided with the same quantity and quality of medical care, there is *vertical equity* in the delivery system. Most geographic research focuses on horizontal equity, but often, both viewpoints are complementary (Meade and Earickson, 2000).

The most basic trade-off is between money and services which arises from the conflict between efficiency and equity in planning and resource allocation. From a geographical perspective, there are important implications. The ultimate aim is to bridge the gap between *access* and *utilisation* of resources; to find the *actual* link between the two. Access to health care is the product of four sets of variables: the *availability* of services, the *possession* of the means of access (money, insurance, transportation etc.), the *non-discriminatory attitudes* of health care providers, and the *failure of the ill themselves* to cope with their situation, such as their ability to recognise symptoms, communicate with health professionals, and navigate the health care system (Meade and Earickson, 2000).

Different disciplinary perspectives have different approaches to utilisation, as outlined by Gatrell (2002); the *sociocultural* approach emphasises factors such as family structure, religion, economic status, health beliefs, and friendship networks. *Sociodemographic* studies deal with population characteristics such as age, sex, education, occupation, ethnicity, and health status. The *social-psychological* approach focuses on knowledge, beliefs, and attitudes about disease and health care. Those who take the *organisational* approach believe that utilisation is mainly determined by the structure of the health services system; they look at things such as government policies and payment plans. The *social systems* approach attempts to fuse the other approaches by considering health care as a system with various components and interrelationships. Much of the present book is an attempt to consider the connections between a *social systems* and an *organisational* approach; in a way that unpacks how the interrelationships and components of a social system feed into organisational systems. The following section shall identify the theoretical approach which grounds this perspective.

Another key geographical issue of health care resource distribution is *scale*. Scale is most simply thought of as the amount of area being considered, from the nation to the neighbourhood, while realising that the area under consideration is at once a component of a larger area and is itself made up of smaller areas: space is a continuum. The word itself originates from the Latin word for ladder, which was both a means of ascent and descent and a set of marks used for measuring (Meade and Earickson, 2000). At the *macroscale* approach to health care management, states have developed their own mathematical calculations using population and deprivation indicators as to how best to achieve equity, such as the *Resource Allocation Working Party* in Britain in the mid-1970s for example. These mathematical models have become increasingly more sophisticated such as that used in Canada, and are based on a variety of measures, including number and type of physicians, population structure, socio-economic status of the area, availability of housing and facilities for physicians, and the area's health needs and resources (Anderson and Rosenberg, 1990). However, this tradition of adopting an essentially positivistic approach often misses the point that the spatial organisation of health care systems cannot be divorced from the political and social context (Meade and Earickson, 2000). Ireland has yet to aspire to a formula based regional allocation strategy (Bond and Conniffe, 2002), favouring political mechanisms and historical continuity for funding allocations to health regions that allow for the corresponding regional needs. Equity is an elusive entity, hard to measure, let alone achieve (Bond and Conniffe, 2002). If it is pursued via formulae alone, it is very difficult to undercover meanings behind data and to investigate consumer needs, perceptions and attitudes of health care, or the role of community groups. Also things like discretionary choices by physicians can be a considerable source of variation, and by its nature is hard to quantify. Therefore, quantitative metrics often miss these nuances on the ground.

At the *meso-scale,* research has demonstrated that 'contextual' variations in health and health care persist from one region of the country to another (Diez-Roux, 2001; MacIntyre et al. 1993). These studies provide insights that show how conditions in particular places are thought to influence health and health related behaviour. Much of the early research concentrated on exploring whether places do indeed 'matter' for health variation and the extent to which they produce significant health inequalities. In retrospect, according to Cummins et al. (2007), this analytical focus has had the unintended consequence of constructing places and people (or 'context' and 'composition') as mutually exclusive and competing explanations for health inequality. Instead, they argue that research needs to focus on the interconnections between people and place in understanding regional variation in health and health care.

Finally, *microscale* studies are often the preferred approach to analysing resource location factors; at the micro-level, the actual mechanisms behind resource distribution decisions are clearer (Meade and Earickson, 2000). The purpose of such analyses is usually to highlight some inequity in spatial distribution, such as rural versus urban. In a study in Canada for example, it was found that doctors, regardless of rural or urban location, ranked spousal influence to be the most important factor when making practice location decisions (Gatrell, 2002).

In a locational sense, the tensions between *efficiency* and *effectiveness* essentially create the spatial properties of health care resources (i.e. *where* the providers are and why they are there). For instance, whether one should provide a single large site or facility (such as a hospital that offers a comprehensive range of services) or provide several smaller facilities that are closer to the population that needs them (Gatrell, 2002) has obvious spatial consequences. There is evidence that people living further away from clinics consult less than those living closer, even when socio-economic status is allowed for; in other words, it is not because of a lack of need that those living further away consult less frequently (Gatrell, 2002). It is also widely assumed that the principal of the 'inverse care law' still applies – that is that primary care services are less available and accessible in areas with the highest levels of need for them. Studies have found that the inverse care law is by no means a universal law that is generalisable to all aspects of primary care provision or indeed applies equally to all sources of population. According to the National Primary Care Research and Development Centre (2005), the strongest evidence of inverse care was found for populations with high concentrations of elderly people and ethnic minorities rather than materially deprived populations per se. The key question is whether geographical 'variation' in the provision and use of health services also represents 'inequity'.

Beyond the basic relationship between consumer and provider, many actors become involved in shaping the equity in the provision or availability of care services. Health care providers can facilitate or hinder the provision of services, and government and the courts are often called on to set policy and adjudicate conflicts between consumers, providers, and financial managers. Political environments inevitably shape health and social programs. Some programmes have become so ingrained as basic benefits that it would be detrimental to tamper with them overtly (Redden, 2002). At the same time, basic philosophic stances can change. For example, the public's view of the appropriate role of government has changed over time and across countries. Some continue to look to government as a means of addressing social programs; others view government as too cumbersome an instrument to function efficiently and expect better results from the private sector.

The former prefer a more paternalistic approach and argue that it is impossible to maintain the principle of equity under a privately operated system of care unless there is at least some adequate level of regulatory oversight. The latter would press for putting more control of one's destiny into one's own hands (under the principle that everyone has an equal opportunity and hence equal responsibility for one's future). However, it is clear that health services require collective action, whether organised publicly or privately, to become individually affordable for everyone. Much of the rhetoric today is directed at identifying the appropriate role for government and the extent to which governmental programmes should continue to be viewed as entitlements.

In practice, England, the US and Ireland fall between the broad perspectives and trends discussed in this chapter. The case study chapters draw from this discussion and examine how the rise of citizenship rights, models of welfare and the shadow state specifically developed in each country. In particular, the case studies trace the rights and welfare entitlements that have been accorded to carers in each country. Central to this is an acknowledgement of geographical variations in the delivery of these entitlements; and a consideration of regional administration structures and the role they play.

Developing a Theoretical Strategy: Towards a Post-Structuralist Understanding of Care

The final aim of this chapter is to develop a theoretical framework in order to deconstruct or tease apart the concepts of citizenship and welfare, and how they apply to the notion of 'carers' in the remainder of this book. Instead of relying on a composite definition of carers and focusing on 'what they do', the remainder of this book is interested in looking at *how* the identity of 'carers' is created, normalised and sustained and what role citizenship and welfare play in constituting their particular sense of history, affinity and separateness. It goes past an essentialist concept of carer to look at how individuals who care are shaped, not in a passive way, but through living everyday practices through a space, which is as much discursively created as non-discursively. To understand these processes better, this book draws upon 'post'-structural theory to help unpack the continual subjectivity of care and welfare which is continually in process, as a site of disunity, conflict and contradictions, and hence potential political change (Johnston, 1994: 468).

Post-structuralism emerged in the late 1960s, with a background of much political unrest as a result of growing dissatisfaction with the established social order across Europe. It was developed chiefly by such theorists as Derrida and Lacan. They drew on the basic insights of structuralism, notably that of linguistics. What was previously thought a fixed relation between the signifier (written or spoken representation) and the signified (actual meaning), post-structuralists argue are continually breaking apart. This led to the method of *deconstruction,* which was Derrida's (1991) method for destabilising claims of 'truth', showing different interpretations and readings.

The poststructuralist analysis of welfare hinges on two key terms – *power*, and the political nature of *knowledge*. These two concepts draw much of their inspiration from Michel Foucault whose ideas were derived in large measure from his analysis of some of the key institutions of the welfare state, in particular, prisons and asylums. Although there are strong elements of structuralism in Michel Foucault's work, such as the deep structure of language, to Foucault it is not an 'iron cage'; there is always resistance (Ritzer and Goodman, 2003). Moreover, his analysis of discourse focuses on the multiple, open-ended, heterogeneous trajectories of discourses, practices, and events, and of establishing their patterned relationships, without recourse to regimes of truth (Ritzer and Goodman, 2003).

One example of the disciplinary society which Foucault proposes comes from *Madness and Civilisation* (Foucault, 1982) where he investigated the historical development of the treatment of those considered 'mad' in the past. Prior to the nineteenth century, 'madness' was not distinguished in any particular way from idleness, infirmity, destitution or delinquency: all represented categories of persons unwilling, or unable, to live within the bounds of the social order. Through the medicalisation and the application of 'psy' knowledges, the 'mad' were dispersed into more specialised institutions which reclassified and reorganised their supervision and treatment. Foucault contests the idea that contemporary 'enlightened' systems for controlling and administering madness represent the substitution of humane treatment for barbaric containment or banishment. He felt that it was simply a result of an epistemic shift in systems of knowledge and control going on in broader mainstream society. Foucault's main point is that embedding 'Reason' in the mundane operations of modern institutions was (and is) framed within the development of an elaborate apparatus of 'unreason' including a multitude of institutions and agencies, a system of assessment and evaluation and rules for the treatment of those judged to be mad. The late twentieth century counterpart shows a similar shift in power relations from the segregated institution to a framework of even smaller modern facilities. However, Foucault (1979; 1982) would argue that 'assessment' and 'judgement' are now undertaken by a different set of social actors – social workers, psychologists, teachers and supervisors, as well as members of the judiciary.

While there is a strong element of structuralism in this work, what is important is that Foucault's attention was directed in particular towards the analysis of forms of truth. For him subjectivity is situated within and transformed by discursive flows, institutional practices and 'games of truth' (Ritzer and Goodman, 2003). What is central to these analyses is not the binary division between 'good' modern practice and 'bad' historical practice, but the reorganisation in the power-relations that sustain our definitions of what is normal and what is abnormal and how these should be treated (O'Brien and Penna, 1998: 119).

A crucial point in Foucault's analysis is that power is not simply imposed in a repressive way from above by the state but it also comes 'from below' and 'from within', through families, social groups, and various types of institutions. The discourses operating within these settings serve to shape the views that people take themselves. The diversity of these discourses means that there are always elements of opposition to the prevailing power relations within places (Pinch, 1997: 118). In the area of public health, much of this control or power is exercised, not through repression but, as Foucault demonstrated, has been created through expert knowledges about human beings which serve to channel thinking and action (Petersen and Lupton, 1996). Because of this 'embedding' of reason, people exercise self-governance, by regulating themselves in the way they think and act. While there are acts of transgression by individuals at every level of society, at the same time there is a moral authority that guides expectations, shapes rules of engagement, and effects ways in which individuals act. In reality, carers' struggles take multiple and diverse forms in everyday local contexts. Their individual struggles over exploitation are an ever-present experience with significant (though not unidirectional) transformative effects (Gibson-Graham, 1996).

Theorising carers' identity in such a way can enable an approach where there is partial identification of social subjects around carer issues and the formulation of strategic solidarities and alliances to effect carer transformation. Importantly though, the book is always aware that these solidarities are discursively as well as nondiscursively constructed and that a carer 'identity' is constructed in the individual social subject by many other discourses of identity and social differentiation. In the words of Mouffe (2005), 'the "identity" of such a multiple and contradictory subject is therefore always contingent and precarious, temporarily fixed at the intersection of those subject positions and dependent on specific forms of identification' (p. 77).

Foucault's emphasis on discourse as an object of enquiry allows us to ask questions not just about experiences and events, but also about the way problems are framed as problems, the way expertise and authority are constructed. Central to this is the notion of 'truth' and how power and knowledge construct such a concept. The research therefore draws on Foucault's analysis of interlocking discursive regimes. It does not reduce political power to the actions of the State; instead it draws attention to the variety of forces and groups that have, in diverse ways, sought to regulate the lives of people, in this case, individual carers.

In the same way, the idea of 'carers' could be seen as something constructed. Post-structuralists (e.g., Derrida, 1991; Delanty, 2000) argue that although these differences are marked, they have no essential existence in and of themselves, but are the products of power-knowledge relationships. Despite the material work of carers being very real, the ways that they are portrayed in societies, and the calls for rights that they invoke are all constructed by power-knowledge relationships between individuals, representative groups, various health professionals, the state and so on. Acknowledging this does not negate any attempt to study them; on the contrary, examining the processes which form and re-form their identity gives a much richer understanding of the broader social and political systems at work.

In these negotiations, 'difference' serves as the vehicle for the distribution of statuses, rights, entitlements, and obligations. The social and political systems through which these distributions are routed constitute the inequalities that differences represent. They comprise the erection and policing of boundaries, borders, limits, inclusions and exclusions, demarcating access to and control over the cultural and social resources that define insider and outsider locations: who is heard and listened to, who defines, legitimates or validates struggles for opportunities and life-chances. Differences are always politicised; they are effects or dimensions of power relations, contesting in every particular arena of struggle for rights, benefits, and social identities (O'Brien and Penna, 1998: 123).

This idea of a politicised identity is very different to an individuals' personal identity. A personal identity does not remain stable, fixed or unified, across the lifecourse and is multiply constructed across different, often intersecting and antagonistic discourses, practices and sites (Isin and Wood, 1999). At the same time however, carers can, as often as not, feel so strongly about their identities and invoke essentialist notions in their struggles for recognition. However the difference is more a false contradiction in the reality of the social world; in the everyday experiences of carers, there are no straightforward boundaries. The institutionalisation of a permanent carers' organisation capable of representing all carers tends to create more durable, recognisable and visible group boundaries. However it is inevitably through the creation of a leading discourse, through mobilising, acting, and organising where the essentialised notion of identity arises.

Given the criticisms of post-structuralist theory for being too exclusionary when every effort of group identification is criticised for essentialism (see Epstein, 1995), it must be stated that to acknowledge the political identity of carers does not mean essentialising them; it means that it is recognised that certain identities are built as durable dispositions via practices which should be used as resources rather than differences to be effaced (Isin and Wood, 1999). It is arguable that some durable dispositions are more 'durable' than others. While all carers are not women, care is still depicted very heavily along these gendered lines for example. At the same time, it is unexceptional for women in most parts of the world to hold jobs outside of the home, yet they still continue to dominate in caregiving jobs and participate in the labour force in ways that differ from men. For this reason, studies of care and labour will continue to appear in feminist literature, alongside notions of patriarchy and gender difference.

In addition, geographers recognise that these durable dispositions can become 'fixed' in space. For example, Wilton's work (1998) on the location of AIDS victims, showed how neighbours felt uncomfortable by the visible presence of patients, and resorted to 'Not In My Back Yard' (NIMBY) community opposition, despite knowing the non-contagious nature of the disease. The process of distancing the 'Other' by spatial partitioning perhaps shows that contemporary lived space could be understood to be an active process of distancing oneself from what we perceive as the 'Other'. Despite these efforts at boundary maintenance however, post-structuralist geographers (see Bhabba 1994; Soja, 1996) argue that the meanings of spaces also change and can be contested by different interests. In short, Foucault's work has been especially influential in terms of developing a recognition of the plurality of knowledge leading to the idea of *geographies*, rather than *the* geography of a subject.

Post-structuralism also enables a more detailed assessment of the role which welfare programmes play in shaping the conditions of emergence, maintenance and contestation of specific identities. Foucault drew attention to the ways in which the history of social policy and welfare is continually made and re-made through discursive and institutional struggles over classification and categorisation of social identities. For struggles to be recognised by citizenship rights, many groups have to compete against each other, as the provisions and status given by rights are subject to change. For carers, what might be available one year may be curtailed the next, and if another excluded group becomes better 'politicised' in mainstream society, the fixed resources must be fought for among the other dependent groups, in effect robbing one to feed the other.

This approach thus instantly allows the recognition of the diversity of welfare institutions for carers. It also enables an analysis of the civil sector, which is regularly in struggles with the state. The implementation and provision of welfare is therefore decentred and distributed throughout the social and institutional networks of the modern political order. In this way, power is not the sole province of the state or capitalist ruling class. Certainly, the state plays a major role in enacting legislation, providing funds through taxation, and establishing targets and goals for the resolution of variously defined 'social problems'. Yet, in many ways, the systems of power described by Foucault are instituted not by openly coercive or repressive state agencies but by a very wide miscellany of civil institutions, such as the Catholic Church in Ireland, as evidenced later in the book.

In terms of a theoretical framework for understanding the remainder of this book, the post-structuralist concept of society as a complex of discourses and institutions or subsystems, each of which performs an indispensable function in maintaining an acceptable degree of societal stability, forms the backdrop to the empirical research. Each societal institution – such as the family, the polity, religion – present environmental norms and values and also constitute sources of resistance on the regime's overall epistemology. Many of the positions, policies, programmes, and procedures of modern organisations are enforced by public opinion, by the views of important constituents, by knowledge legitimated through the educational system, by social prestige, by the laws, and by the definitions of negligence and caution used by the courts (Donnelly-Cox and O'Regan, 1998). Such elements of formal structure are manifestations of powerful and rationalised discourses that are binding on particular social groups.

The discursive regulatory regimes in each international case study chapter shall serve as a common tie to compare across states; to see how the power-knowledge discourses play out in the field of welfare for carers and their care recipients. It is apparent that each welfare system is not simply ruled by a top-down *power* in the negative sense of the word. Rather, the discursive and material practices of resistance and regulation continuously inform and bring change to the governmental and voluntary system. This approach shall apply to each case-study chapter, comparing England, the US, and Ireland. Part III deviates from this to see how carers themselves are grounded within one such regulatory regime; that of Ireland. It examines the discursive and material practices of carers by investigating the modes of regulation, resistance and influence that take place at this scale. This facilitates an examination of what it is like for individuals to live 'as carers', in a site where their identity is created and normalised through citizenship, welfare, and social conceptions of gender and class. It is possible to see how their particular sense of affinity and separateness is shaped by these outside discourses, and how at the same time, individuals through everyday struggles, make their own transformative effects.

PART II
Comparative Perspectives in the Development of care

Chapter 4
Carer's Policy in England

This chapter explores and identifies what was historically specific about England, in terms of its carer policy as echoed through its welfare state. It builds on the earlier chapter by examining the formation of rights for carers and persons with disabilities by the British state. The British model of welfare is, as Esping-Andersen notes, a rather uneasy mix of universalism and the market (1990). Its present health and welfare system is a classic example of an early fully nationalised system of support and care provision that has undergone many transitions towards a neo-liberal system of care (see timeline in Table 4.1 overleaf). This chapter details the progression of ideas and discourses of care through this period and examines the emergence of informal caring in today's context.

The Development of Welfare and Social Services

The first consolidated attempt at state 'care policy' was the *Poor Law Act* 1601. This made provision for a compulsory poor rate to be levied on every parish, the creation of 'overseers' of relief, and the collection of a poor relief rate from property owners (Bloy, 2002). One common means of local support for disabled people, then was direct support to the family involved, in the form of either straightforward cash payments or allocations of food and other supplies from the common stock kept by many communities for just such purposes (Ferguson, 2004). The state held a suspicion of people claiming charity and the 'overseers' provided a way of controlling the 'lower orders'[1] and reinforced a sense of social hierarchy. Two types of relief were available; outdoor relief, where the dependents would be left in their own homes and would be given either a 'dole' of money on which to live or be given relief in kind – clothes and food, for example. The care of people with disabilities was characterised by a tolerance of care in the home by society as long as they were not of the 'wandering' poor (Bloy, 2002). Porter (1992) says that detailed studies of English rural communities as late as the 17th and 18th centuries have shown that families aided by parish poor relief were still typically expected to assume the role of looking after their disabled relatives at home. However, such studies also found people hidden away in a cellar or in a barn, or in the case of the more affluent, under the care of the servants.

1 Throughout this book, original terminology of the times as found in policy and legislation are used to denote the changing discourses around disability.

Table 4.1 English Disability and Care Legislation

Discourse	Act of Legislation	Purpose of Legislation
Promotion of Institutional Care. Punitive view of dependency and disability.	*1601 Poor Law Act*	Established indoor relief in almshouses and outdoor relief in their own homes with a 'dole' of money on which to live or be given relief in kind – clothes and food, for example.
	1744 Vagrancy Act	Made the first distinction between paupers and lunatics and made some provision for the treatment of care of lunatics from parish relief funds. This saw the growth of privately owned institutions across the country known as 'madhouses'.
	1828 Madhouse Act	Established a stricter regime of licensing and visiting committees for asylums.
	1834 Poor Law Amendment Act	Made a fundamental alteration which prohibited outdoor relief. This made it both convenient from an administrative point of view and provided a financial incentive at local authority level which further helped push up numbers admitted to asylums.
	1845 Lunatics Act	Established the asylum system as the proper and primary system for the treatment of lunacy, making it compulsory for each county to provide an asylum within three years of its passing.
	1886 Idiots Act	Required that authorities establish asylums for the care, education and training of the 'mentally retarded'.
	1890 Lunacy Act	Was seen as copper fastening this custodial approach. Asylums became more like regimented custodial holding centres.
	1913 Mental Deficiency Act	Both promoted institutional care, but also set up a system of care in the community. Three types of formal care were created – institutional care, guardianship, and supervision.
	1927 Mental Deficiency Act	Made it a duty of local authorities to provide training for 'defectives', through occupation centres.
	1930 Mental Treatment Act	Recommended the care of mental illness along modern public health lines, still endorsed involuntary certification and the use of force to place a patient to an asylum.

Created ‘deserving’ and ‘non-deserving’ distinction between disabled people.	*1944 Disabled Persons (Employment) Act*	Accommodated disabled ex-soldiers in the search for work. Did not focus on non-soldier adults like those with intellectual disabilities.
Reconstruction of society after the War. Re-enforced traditional family roles.	*1944 Social Insurance Act*	Beveridge’s new Welfare Payments System.
	1948 National Assistance Act	Created duties and powers for authorities to provide care homes and community care services. Under section 42, a man is liable to maintain his wife. And, a woman is liable to maintain her husband. This meant that where a person’s accommodation is provided at the public expense by a local authority, the local authority may ask the liable relative to refund all or part of that expenditure.
	1948 NHS Act	Established the National Health Service, which was to become the Model of Health Care in the UK.
Normalisation and Social Role Valorisation, leading to first acknowledgement of need for community care.	*1959 Mental Health Act*	Repealed all the Lunacy and Mental Treatment Acts from 1890 to 1930, and the Mental Deficiency Acts, 1913 to 1938, and made fresh provision with respect to the treatment and care of ‘mentally disordered’ persons.
	1970 Chronically Sick and Disabled Persons Act	Specified services which Local Authorities should provide for disabled people. It stated that the Social Services Department must assess the disabled person’s need for the provision of or assistance in obtaining services.
	1970 Education (Handicapped Children) Act	Transferred education services for children with a learning disability from health to local authorities.
	1970 Local Authority Social Services Act	Gave local authorities responsibility for the development of social work departments, whose functions were to include that of community care.

Table 4.1 continued

First acknowledged mothers and daughters as 'carers'.	*1975 Social Security Act*	Established the Invalidity Care Allowance for Carers (currently Carers Allowance)
	1980 Social Security Act	Cut the link between the value of social security benefits like the flat rate 'basic' state pension and measures of other incomes or earnings.
	1986 Disabled Persons Act	Promoted the identification and assessment of disabled school leavers to avoid service dislocation and to develop long-term perspectives of individual and family needs. The Local Authority had to have regard for a carer's ability to continue to provide care on a regular basis when the needs of the disabled person were being assessed.
	1989 Children Act	Established new divisions in health and social services agencies along the lines of purchasers and providers in both sectors. It also confirmed divides between adults and children in social services.
Decided that health and community care should be separate.	*1990 National Health Service and Community Care Act* (1993 when fully implemented)	Assigned responsibility for assessing needs and putting together packages of care to meet those needs to local authority. The passage of this Act can be considered as a 'defining moment' in the acceptance of care within communities as the preferred way of meeting the needs of disabled people.
	1991 Disability Living Allowance & Disability Working Allowance Act	Introduced the 'disability living allowance' (DLA) for those who received the middle or highest rate care and 'disability working allowance' (DWA).
Acknowledgement of the value and importance of the work that carers do.	*1995 Carers (Recognition and Services) Act*	Legally recognised the term 'carer'. Gave the local authority the duty to carry out an assessment on carers' needs.
Recognised disability as a rights issue rather than charity.	*1995 Disability Discrimination Act*	Gave disabled people new rights in the areas of employment, access to goods and services and buying or renting land or property.

	1996 Community Care (Direct Payments) Act	Enabled local authorities responsible for community care services to make payments direct to people, enabling them to arrange the services themselves.
	1999 NHS Act	Combined into a single budget the resources previously held in separate funding streams for hospital and community health services.
	2000 Carers and Disabled Children Act.	Enabled local councils to make direct payments to parents of disabled children and to disabled 16 to 17 year-olds but will also required local authorities to pay attention to the needs of parent carers and to any barriers to social inclusion that face the whole family.
	2003 Community Care Act	Improved carers' rights to ensure their needs are addressed before a patient is considered 'safe for discharge'.
Carers become a fundamental national concern.	*2004 Carers (Equal Opportunities) Act*	Ensured that carers now have to be told about their rights, have more opportunities for work, education and leisure and there will be greater collaboration between statutory services to help them in their caring roles.
Broadening of Disability Rights.	*Disability Discrimination Act 2005*	Made substantial amendments to the Disability Discrimination Act 1995. The DDA represents a new approach. It focuses on institutional change rather than adjustments for individuals.

There was also indoor relief, where disabled persons would be taken into a local poorhouse (workhouse). The poorhouse from the beginning was the acknowledged last resort for the most troublesome or severely disabled cases (Ferguson, 2004). The Poor Law was administered at the parish level in England. There were 15,000 parishes throughout England and Wales, each based on a parish church, however no mechanism was introduced to enforce any of the measures stated by the 1601 Act and the operation of the poor law was inconsistent. The legislation did not set down any administrative standards so parishes were at liberty to interpret the law in any way they wished (Bloy, 2002).

In 1744 the *Vagrancy Act* made the first distinction between paupers (extremely poor) and lunatics (those with mental illness) and made some provision for the treatment of care of lunatics from parish relief funds. This saw the growth of privately owned institutions across the country known as 'madhouses' and 'idiot asylums' (for those with intellectual disabilities). This movement owed little to any tangible medical breakthroughs, but perhaps offered some solution to the problems of industrialisation and pauperisation. At the same time, the *Madhouse Act* (1744) required that madhouses be licensed. Rogers and Pilgrim (2001) argue that the 'great confinement' (as described by Foucault), which occurred in France never happened in England where the landscape of care was much more fragmented consisting of a range of non-institutionalised and private options (Goodwin, 1997).

The state began to take more interest in asylums in the nineteenth century. At this time, insane persons were chargeable to their respective parishes in Gaols, Houses of Correction, Poor Houses and Houses of Industry. The *County Asylum Act* (1808) regarded this *ad hoc* practice as inconvenient, thus counties were given powers to construct State Asylums. The *Madhouse Act* (1823) established a stricter regime of licensing and visiting committees for asylums (Roberts, 2001). According to Scull (1993), 'more and more the asylum was presented as a technical, objective, scientific response to the patient's condition, an environment which provided the best possible conditions for his recovery'.

The *Poor Law Amendment Act* (1834), made a fundamental alteration to the *Poor Law* which prohibited outdoor relief. This had major implications for family carers, however despite efforts to ban outdoor relief, parishes often continued to offer it as a more cost effective method of dealing with pauperism. Despite much opposition, this Act formed the basis of poor relief throughout the country for over a century. It replaced the earlier haphazard parish level approach with a highly centralised system which encouraged the large scale development of workhouses by Poor Law Unions. It was supplemented by the *Lunatics Act* (1845) which established the asylum system as the proper and primary system for the treatment of lunacy, making it compulsory for each county to provide an asylum within three years of its passing. Prior to this legislation, asylums had differed markedly in size and quality of care. Many different explanations have been cited for the development of this elaborate system of asylum care. Firstly, it was seen to have been a result of the spread of Enlightenment thinking, where the application of scientific reason could offer solutions to society's problems and difficulties. Secondly, it was argued that the rise of industrialisation which led to the transition from agriculture and cottage-based industries to 'waged-based' systems demarcated disabled people as less-productive (Oliver and Barnes, 1998; Gleeson, 1999).

While these institutions were largely lunacy asylums, there was also a large amount of 'idiots' in their care. Thus, in 1847, a small group of medical practitioners and nonconformist philanthropists led by the Congregationalist Minister Andrew Reed established a charitable asylum designed specifically for idiots, first in London and later in a large purpose-built asylum in Surrey – the 'National Asylum for Idiots' (later, Earlswood Asylum) (Wright, 2004). John Langdon Down, one of the premier practitioners in England, advocated the creation of idiot institutions separate from lunatic asylums, with the perceived benefit of classification and specialised treatment.

The process of exclusion thus became more complex and sophisticated with an equal rise in professional dominance (eg. jobs in psychology, medicine, nursing care) in the process. In 1857, legislation, as a matter of course, required the medical certification of idiots and lunatics. The spread of 'psychiatry' in British medicine from the mid-nineteenth century made it clear that medical authority should take precedence and the new compulsory asylums were now to be run by medical practitioners (Scull, 1993). Administrating control therefore was only valid if a medical 'expert' was in charge. Much of the early psychological profession however believed that madness and idiocy were actually caused by defective and/or careless families, thus leading to their proper 'moral treatment' in asylums (Jones, 2002).

Philo (1987) has drawn attention to the way people with disabilities were 'cared for', in particular, mental patients in England. He was interested in looking at how asylums were considered normal and 'natural' for people with mental illness as they were removed from the normal round of people and places in a society. In the following excerpt from the *Transactions of the Association for the Promotion of Social Science* (c. 1850), one can see the way the 'caring' profession saw it fit to remove the patient from 'all the influences and all the associations' of the home;

> It seems to have been too much forgotten that in every case of insanity the first object should be, as in other maladies, the recovery of the patient: and that is often impossible without *a removal of the patient from home*. All the influences and all the associations of home become perverted, in the large majority of cases, in this unhappy malady (cited in Philo, 1987: 402) (my emphasis).

Home care by default was portrayed as a poor site of care. From the above quote, it is also possible to identify the medicalisation of care. In the wake of Darwin's *Origins of the Species*, physicians became drawn to the implications of evolutionary theory to ethnology. 'Idiots' became associated with the Mongolian race and it was argued that individuals could 'revert' from one racial type to another 'premodern' race. This culminated with the new science of eugenics in the 1880s. The *Idiots Act* (1886) required that authorities establish asylums for the care, education and training of 'idiots'. The *Lunacy Act* (1890) was seen as copper-fastening this custodial approach and consolidated much previous legislation. It also introduced judicial authority for ordering the detention of a person as a lunatic and put restrictions on the opening of new private asylums. Asylums became more like regimented custodial holding centres. Although this came under the guise of 'treatment', the will of the state, the medical professionals, and the general public was to remove those with mental illness, physical/sensory and intellectual disabilities from society by placing them in institutions so that their disability could be hidden from mainstream society. While many families continued to care in the shadow of the asylum, the rates of those institutionalised confirmed that many more were handed over to the care of the state.

The Early Twentieth Century (1900–1940)

England's care policy in the beginning of the twentieth century was marked most clearly by the passing of the *Mental Deficiency Act* (1913). It gave Hospital Boards of Governors extensive powers to prevent the discharge from hospital of any patient they deemed unfit for release. Once admitted through the 'certification' process, discharge back into society was often long delayed (Dale, 2003). Local authorities were given the duty to ascertain, certify, and institutionalise 'mental defectives' including those with intellectual disabilities. While the Act promoted institutional care, it also set up a system of care in the community; guardianship, and supervision (Roberts, 2001). Guardianship meant that individuals could be placed in the control of a suitable person (parental application had to be accompanied with a certificate signed by two doctors, one of whom was approved for the purpose), and local authorities could provide financial assistance to them (Eldergill, no date). Supervision consisted of the visiting of 'defectives' in their homes by salaried local authority officials, such as health visitors, enquiry officers and district nurses, and also by the members of local voluntary organisations. These visitors prepared quarterly reports for local Mental Deficiency Committees (Bartlett and Wright, 1999). Those families that had a member who had been certified were subject to regular scrutiny from officials for their ability to both care for, and control them. In particular, families were asked by visitors about their ability to prevent 'defectives' from associating with the opposite sex. Families were scrutinised when decisions were made about discharges from institutions, home leave from institutions, and in regard to suitability for licensing (Walmsley and Rolph, 2001). In addition, the subsequent *Mental Deficiency Act* (1927) made it a duty of local authorities to provide training for 'defectives', through occupation centres (Walmsley and Rolph, 2001).

Many individuals did remain with their families, who retained some influence over them. For example, statistics provided by the Board of Control showed that in 1939, there were 46,054 'defectives' in institutions, and 43,850 under statutory supervision (Walmsley and Rolph, 2001). It was often very difficult to resist the pressure to institutionalise though, and local archives tell the stories of mothers writing to asking for their children to be allowed home again (Atkinson, 1997). State control into the family and guardianship was thus very restrictive and families had little autonomy.

As a result of the dual mandate within the *Mental Deficiency Act* (1913) between institutional and community care, there were cases of 'mental defectives' being institutionalised against the wishes of the family, cases of families effectively resisting institutional care, but also cases of families asking for institutional care and being turned down. 'Idiots' or 'imbeciles' (the most profoundly disabled in official terminology of the time) who posed no threat to public order, such as those with Down's syndrome, were particularly likely to be left at home and to receive minimal care (Walmsley, 2001). In the National Sound Archive (2000) there are accounts of people with cerebral palsy and Down's syndrome living at home with their families who were largely ignored by authorities, with services patchy in the extreme and mostly voluntary. The Act in general though greatly increased the number of people with mild learning disabilities (the 'feeble minded') detained in institutions. What also seems clear is that the social status of the family was important in determining what care their 'mentally defective' family members received. In Bedfordshire, it appears that families deemed to be 'respectable' were supported, whereas those where poverty and poor home management was in evidence were more likely to attract greater attention and the prospect of institutionalisation (Rolph and Walmsley, 2006).

It was the outbreak of the First World War that the readiness to compensate became a common principle of England's disability legislation. Between 1914 and 1920, legislation was passed to provide war pensions, to compensate those injured, to help those who had been widowed or orphaned, and to regulate charities for the wounded. However, there was a difference in attitudes between those impaired from the war 'deserving' and those previously disabled 'undeserving' (Powell and Guerin, 1997) as eugenic ideals continued to inform people's beliefs in academic and medical circles (Quin and Redmond, 2005: 149). As Stone (1985) puts it, Victorian psychiatry's theories on mental illness 'was significantly dented as young men of respectable and proven character were reduced to mental wrecks with a few months in the trenches' (p. 245). The *Mental Treatment Act* (1930), although recommending the care of mental illness along modern public health lines, still endorsed involuntary certification and the use of force to place a patient in an asylum.

The 1930s saw the advancement of a more advanced medicalisation of intellectual disability. At the same time, the eugenic acceptance which had developed in the 1880s had by this time surfaced to centre stage in national discourse and State policy. People with intellectual disabilities were viewed as the products of innate family dysfunction. Families were perceived to be variously irresponsible, sexually overactive, poor and criminals. The widely noted book, *The Mongol in Our Midst* (1924), by British physician F.G. Crookshank furthered the view that Mongol ('primitive') blood, which was causing idiocy, no doubt flowed in the veins of many Europeans (Wright, 2004). The *Wood Committee* in the UK (1929) represented the peak of this movement; both segregation and sterilisation were used as explicit attempts to control families and the *Report on Mental Deficiency* of 1929 enabled removal and incarceration under the guise of social protection (Manthorpe, 1994). The period between 1930 and 1936 marked the high point of the sterilisation campaign in Britain (Webster, 2003).

World War Two – Beveridge Welfare State (1940–1949)

The Second World War was another catalyst towards the further development of England's care policy. This was evident in the passing of the *War Charities Act* (1940), the *Determination of Needs Act* (1941) and the *Disabled Persons (Employment) Act* (1944). However, it is possible to discern similar divisive public attitudes and motives at work in this legislation between the war wounded, who were deemed 'unnaturally abnormal', and disabled people as 'naturally abnormal' (Drake, 1999: 50). As a result, people with disabilites found themselves displaced by the priority given to disabled ex-soldiers in the search for work, accommodation and access to health services. Whilst the Poor Law was finally removed from the statute book in 1948, it had nevertheless left a legacy of attitudes and practices redolent of poverty and minimal service.

The War was also a catalyst towards the development of the welfare state proper in England, marked by the *1942 Social Insurance and Allied Services Report (The Beveridge Report)*, which advocated social insurance and universal benefits to alleviate deprivation. It was enshrined in the *Social Insurance Act* (1944). In drafting the report, major consultation took place with trade unions and the voluntary sector. When the war in Europe ended in May 1945, Churchill called a general election for July. Labour's manifesto captured the public mood for change and achieved a landslide victory. The international post-war economic boom allowed Labour to take on Beveridge's proposals and dramatically expand the scope of welfare services.

Beveridge's proposals brought about the creation and growth of social services. While descended from liberal roots, Britain developed a model in which universal benefits and services were substantially expanded by a paternalistic state concerned about the health of its war veterans and workforce beyond minimum levels (George and Taylor-Gooby, 1996). Commentators, such as the RNID charity, have pointed out that the 'insurance' character of the system was always a myth. This was technically correct as payments have been always funded through the general tax system, rather than the National Insurance Fund. However, it was an important ideological strategy to win society-wide support, as insurance was regarded easier to digest than the stigma of pre-war means-tested 'handouts' (RNID, 1999).

The principle of a welfare state was one which – at least in public – all the major political parties in Britain supported in the beginning (Graham, 1999: 288). The prototypical characteristics of it included government dominance in the administrative and fiscal dimensions of health policy-making and implementation, funded by compulsory contributions to general revenue. In the main, although Beveridge made a claim to setting up a universal system of welfare support, his proposals were really designed to fill the gaps where the market and family failed; not to replace them as the main source of support to individuals (Clarke and Langan, 2001a). The expansion was framed by the presumption that most welfare needs would be satisfied by the family and the market (except in education and public health). The Labour government had to maintain a commitment to full-employment in order to finance such a program, and it was assumed that full employment meant full *male* employment. Women were structurally positioned in the benefit system as dependants. The idea of welfare was based on an economic and social architecture in which the 'family wage' was the linchpin, linking the labour market to the distribution of social roles and dependency by age and gender within the family (Clarke and Langan, 2001a). The key economic foundation of the post-war welfare regime was the presumption that a managed economy would deliver full employment as a political objective.

For Beveridge there was to be an increasingly residual role played by a further layer of non-insured benefits, *National Assistance*, where means-testing played a central role (Clarke and Langan, 2001b). These piecemeal compensatory measures gradually expanded and were woven into a more coherent system of social security. Welfare therefore was expressed in the form of pension payments, disability and sickness benefits, a growth in health services, and support for social welfare activities.

State involvement in disabled people's lives also increased steadily throughout this period. From somewhat fragmented beginnings, social work and a refinement of professional interventions in the lives of disabled people developed rapidly and continued to expand through the 1950s and 60s. In addition, there was a significant increase in child care officers, probation officers and medical, psychiatric and social workers who received different training and had separate roles in separate service structures (Drake, 1999: 58). The overriding aim of welfare was to 'rehabilitate' disabled people, and the new professions claimed that they had the expertise necessary for the job.

At the same time, there was a change in the perception of the role of the voluntary sector, from that of a key provider of welfare services to that of supplementary support. Emphasis was placed on the moral contribution that voluntarism had to play in society. As a consequence, voluntarism continued to be encouraged through local and central government grant-aid. Councils for Voluntary Service, CVS, for example, were local voluntary organisations set up and run by local groups to support, promote and develop local voluntary action. In 1945 CVS linked up to form a national network, called the National Association of Councils for Voluntary Service. As such, voluntary organisations reoriented their services in order to differentiate their contribution to welfare support from that of the state (Scorfield, 1999).

Families also became more involved as members of voluntary efforts, as well as early pressure groups for improved services. They began, in the late 1940s and 1950s, individually to challenge professional and public attitudes and the actions (or inaction) or local authorities, and to take steps towards change. This resulted in the formation of voluntary organisations such as the *National Association of Parents of Backward Children (NAPBC)* in 1946, later known as *Mencap*, one of the largest grass-roots voluntary movements to be formed in postwar Britain. This organisation pushed local authorities to establish services such as respite care, residential homes and employment opportunities. But above all, families pushed for more and better education in the form of occupation centres, often paid for and run by themselves (Welshman and Walmsey, 2006).

From a geographical point of view the post-war reconstruction of welfare in Britain involved the elaboration of a new set of relationships between the state, the market, voluntary sector, and the family thus changing the overall landscape of care. In considering that set of relationships it is useful to think of welfare provision not as a unitary structure ('the welfare state') but as a complex and changing pattern of relationships between the different sectors. In addition, three departments were made responsible for personal social services: health departments, responsible for public health and various aspects of social care; welfare departments, responsible for residential care and support for elderly and disabled people; and children's departments, responsible for child care (Rolph et al., 2006).

Idea of Community Care (1950–1959)

The concept of de-institutionalisation developed during the 1950s and 1960s, largely in response to the prohibitive costs of institutions across the Western world. In addition, the restrictive nature of institutions, the unhealthy living conditions and an increase in reported abuse to members within them also facilitated the endorsement by governments of this course of action. The process entailed the closure and/or downscaling of institutions and their replacement by a variety of community-care options. However, in the 1950s the term 'carer' did not figure in either research or policy. In a chapter titled 'The Family System of Care', Townsend (1957) focused on the *family* rather than *individuals* as the cornerstone of care, yet at the same time, made it quite clear that the care provided by London families of the 1950s fell primarily on women (see Bytheway and Johnson, 2008).

Some of the first changes in public policy towards a community approach can be seen in the *Report of the Royal Commission on the Law Relating to Mental Illness and Mental Deficiency* in 1957, which stated, 'we are convinced that the aim should be a deliberate re-orientation away from residential care in its present form and towards residential homes in the community' (Royal Commission, 1957). It also argued that local authority community services should be available to all who needed them and that formal 'ascertainment' could be dispensed with: 'the whole approach should be a positive one offering help and obtaining the co-operation of the patient and his family' (Royal Commission, 1957, p, 101, para. 294). An important principle was that, where possible, patients should make use of general services. There was a shift in emphasis from hospitals to community care: it was not 'in the best interests of patients' that they should live for long periods in large or remote institutions, cut off from the 'normal' worlds and from mixing with other people (Royal Commission, 1957, p. 207, para. 601).

Its legislative counterpart, the *1959 Mental Health Act,* repealed all the *Lunacy and Mental Treatment Acts* from 1890 to 1930, and the *Mental Deficiency Acts*, 1913 to 1938, and made fresh provision with respect to the treatment and care of 'mentally disordered' persons (Roberts, 2001). It laid the basis for community care services such as training and occupation centres, social centres and clubs, home visiting services, and residential homes and hostels. Thus, the emphasis on care provision was increasingly being reoriented *away* from institutions to community care (Drake, 1999: 54). However, while the Royal Commission was highly significant, its commitment was not matched by its legislative counterpart, the *1959 Mental Health Act*, which failed to make provision of local authority services compulsory, or make financial provision for additional capital expenditure (Busfield, 1986). Amongst the services delivered by the post-war welfare state, community care ranked low in terms of public expenditure levels (Webb and Wistow 1986, cited in Lewis 1999).

Despite this, asylum rates began to drop. This was largely to do with changing patterns of admission and discharge of people with intellectual disabilities and the elderly. The government sought to sustain disabled people in the community using vocational training, sheltered workshops and other services. At the time however, there was a failure to develop community-based alternatives that would reduce the *need* for individuals to enter institutional care (Seebohm Report: Cm. 3703, 1968). Waiting lists for day and residential services for people with intellectual and physical disabilities, along with a shortage of domiciliary services were evident in many areas across England.

Expansion and Retrenchment (1960–1978)

The increase in State interest in community care at the start of the 1960s was instigated by right-wing civil libertarians like former Minister for Health, Enoch Powell, dubbed by some the Father of Community Care, who argued that mental hospitals were effectively prisons, preventing a return to normal life (BBC News, 1999). In terms of the discourse of care at the time, the concept of 'Normalisation', first articulated by Bengt Nirje (1969), became used by community care advocates. It was defined as the principle by which people with a disability have the right to lead a valued ordinary life, based on the belief in their equality as human beings and citizens (Ramon, 1991). It became a concept community care proponents used to question the ethical basis for institutionalisation. The term has since become synonymous with the work of Wolf Wolfensberger with his normalisation model, and subsequently articulated as social role valorisation (SRV). Wolfensberger felt that normalisation would be achieved when those with intellectual disabilities acquired personal and vocational skills which would enable them to live lives as normal as possible through employment, ordinary housing and access to non-segregated leisure pursuits. This movement was given a major endorsement by the state's focus on the rationalisation of the asylum system (Wearing, 1998). However, the transformation effort required an enormous and continued commitment by government and theories of normalisation and SRV helped sustain this commitment; it thus had a major impact on disability policy and service developments in England, as well as the United States, since the 1960s and 70s (Wearing, 1998).

Community care emerged in policy discourse with *The Seebohm Report 1968* which is generally considered a watershed in the development of community-based services for disabled people living at home. It advocated the introduction of social services departments within local authorities. It highlighted the need for more effective co-ordination between social services, housing, health, education and social security, in order to support such policies. It recommended the setting up of a unitary social services department to take over the work of the existing three separate departments (health, welfare, children) within the local authority structure to meet the social needs of the community. This gave the impetus to social work as a generic profession, though genericism is increasingly rare in practice. In the report, Seebohm referred to a wider conception of social service, not directed only to the care of social casualties but to the whole community. The personal social services therefore were encouraged to see themselves as part of a network of services within the community and to assist the growth of community identity and mutual aid to combat social problems (Bulmer, 1987). This was a significant step towards social work for family carers looking after people with disabilities.

With the rise of government focus on community care, and in response to Seebohm's report, social service departments (SSDs) were set up in 1970 in each local authority, under the *Local Authority Social Services Act*. This gave local authorities the responsibility for the development of these departments, whose functions were to include that of community care. There are nearly 200 local authorities in England, ranging from enormous counties like Lancashire and huge conurbations like Birmingham to small unitary authorities like Rutland and the Corporation of London. The professional issues facing social services directors in Kent and Rutland are similar, but the management task is very different. Indeed, the major local authority areas in England contained the largest populations under local authority control in the Western World at this time (Douglas and Philpot, 1998). This reorganisation had a major geographical impact on the ground. According to Harbert and Rogers (1983) the Director of Social Services in one authority, Avon, observed that when SSDs were created, it became apparent that statutory services were not able to meet all the demands from a sophisticated and articulate public. Self-help groups were useful but had limitations, needing access to skills and financial resources outside the scope of their members. A more community-based approach was therefore developed in which social service departments identified needs and went out into the community to locate the skills and other resources required to meet them by seeking out resources in the community and, when necessary, providing training and expert back-up services (Bulmer, 1987: 5). The Act also gave local authorities a responsibility for establishing a social work committee with responsibilities for (amongst other roles): the provision and regulation of residential accommodation and welfare services for disabled persons – including practical assistance in the home, day centres, visiting and advisory services; and assisting housing authorities in relation to cases of homelessness.

The creation of local authority SSDs focused explicitly on the provision of a 'family service' which positioned the family in a number of different ways. Like other policy domains, it assumed both the normality and desirability of the nuclear family, and aimed to address concerns about 'family failure' by providing social work services to improve family functioning. They were responsible for those who, for one reason or another, were not being cared for by or within families and thus required (or were seen to need) public residential care (Clarke and Langan, 2001b).

The dual function of social services, linking family intervention and care services, put social workers at the forefront of the movement towards 'community care'. The early 1970s saw the start of the run-down of hospitals caring for those with an intellectual disability. However, community care services were very much in their infancy. Ayer and Alaszewski (1984), studying a group of North Humberside mothers who were caring for their children with a learning disability, noted that despite the advocating of community care in the Seebohm report, they could find little evidence of a co-ordinated system of support on the ground for the mothers they talked to. At the heart of community care was an assumption that networks of care would or could be available within the community to provide support (Clarke and Langan, 2001b). This rested on the belief that networks of 'primary carers' rather than professional carers would play the dominant role in providing such support. In that context, primary care was identified with the family (or women) as wives, mothers, daughters and sisters of those who needed care (Clarke and Langan, 2001b).

The expansion of welfare through to the 1970s can be seen as the product of changing patterns of need. Changing demographic patterns affected the level of demands for social as well as health care significantly, ranging from accommodation to personal support (Clarke and Langan, 2001b). The most important benefits in the 'disability' portfolio – Invalidity Benefit and Non-Contributory Invalidity Pension – were introduced in the 1970s when the principles of the post-war insurance scheme were already under severe stress, due to demographic change, fiscal crisis, and increases in unemployment. The net result is that the system of disability payments in England has since been 'extraordinarily complicated' (Leat and Ungerson, 1994: 261). It also influenced the growth of a wider 'welfare rights' movement over the next two decades.

The Disability Rights Movement became more organised and vociferous in the 1970s, and the struggle for self-determination and an end to 'dependency born of powerlessness, poverty, degradation, and institutionalisation' (Charlton, 1998: 3) gathered momentum. Whilst Wolfensberger developed the idea of citizen advocacy – the partnership of a 'valued' person speaking on behalf of a vulnerable person – the self-advocacy movement focused on people speaking for themselves. Rights-based perspectives replaced the traditional needs-based approach linked to the notion of charity, enabling disabled people, and to some extent their families, to retain dignity in demanding rights rather than begging for acts of kindness (Bandman, 1973). By the 1970s the conditions of many institutions caring for those with an intellectual disability had begun to come under public scrutiny. In England, Ryan and Thomas wrote *The Politics of Mental Handicap* (1987) about the degradation suffered by those in mental handicap hospitals. As a result, throughout the 1970s and 1980s, the numbers of people with intellectual disability in institutional care dropped, large institutions closed and care in smaller units and houses based in the community were introduced (Ryan and Thomas, 1987).

At this time, families gained more visible influence where they were organised as part of the advocacy movement. For the first time since welfare policy started in England, attention only began to focus on direct support for informal carers in 1975, when the government introduced the 'Invalid Care Allowance', under the *Social Security Act* (1975). At this time, the family occupied a rather more complex position in relation to state welfare than might have been predicted from the assumptions of 1945. The core presumption of the conventional nuclear family as the cornerstone of social care still prevailed and the assumption of heterosexual cohabitation still dominated social security provision. Until the mid-1980s, the Invalid Care Allowance was not granted to married women caring for a sick or disabled relative on the grounds that this was a part of their normal duties (UK Parliament, 1991). There were growing signs that reality was failing to live up to the ideal nuclear family model, which led government to make pessimistic interpretations of societal changes such as lamenting the loss of the traditional family and obligation on the part of younger generations (Clarke and Langan, 2001b).

The growing gulf between the assumptions made of the nuclear family and the reality of family life placed contradictory demands on social policy. On the one hand, the state provision of care had developed around the assumption that the family would normally provide support for its members and therefore state support would be the exception. As the exceptions increased, there was concern that the very existence of state support itself was producing the deviations from the ideal. This argument is sometimes referred to as the 'perverse incentive' of insurance (Clarke and Langan, 2001b). This realisation of the state not accepting or easing the undue burden placed on families led to a plethora of social theorists like Barnes (1997), Ramon (1991), Parr (1997) and Gleeson and Kearns (2001) to re-appraise community care and critique its assumptions. In general, advocates of community care, including policy makers and academics alike, had assumed a better deal for people with disabilities and their families in society. They were convinced that the readiness of the population to solve problems would increase when the problems were made visible. It was thought that by putting disabled people back into society, that the origins of their marginalisation could be combated.

It was hoped that the relocation from isolated stand-alone institutions would help to get rid of, or diminish stigmatisation, but some researchers such as Thomas (2003), Parr (1997), and Milligan (2000) have refuted this, showing that there was little difference in a person's expectations of stigmatisation as a result of relocating them to the community. The effects of stigma among other things made disabled people, particularly those with mental illness and intellectual disability – a less vocal group in demanding improved conditions. This was a serious impediment when it came to demanding a fair slice of resources in a very competitive environment. Social exclusion continued with many people still exhibiting nervousness, fear, and basic ignorance to people with disabilities. As Christie (1989), an advocate of sheltered villages remarked, community care in ordinary society '…sounds fine, until one looks into that ordinary society' (cited in Gleeson and Kearns, 2001: 67).

In addition to society's slowness to change attitudes, there remained many advocate groups formally linked to institutions or parents whose siblings were patrons of them. For these people, de-institutionalisation represented insecurity, a change from the assurance derived from knowing that one's relative was in lifelong institutional care to the uncertainty of a new and open service regime. This form of opposition also articulated a view of the service user as vulnerable. This was frequently the mirror image of the other paradigm; the normalised (or 'socially valorised') subjectivity, imagined by supporters of community care (Gleeson and Kearns, 2001). Therefore there were two co-existing paradigms in conflict with each other. It appears therefore that neither geographical space nor social attitudes, were fully prepared for the re-entry of people with intellectual disabilities to society.

While the discourse of caregiving was slowly evolving, by and large, the extent of informal caregiving was generally overlooked at this time. The Wolfenden Committee Report (1978) *The Future of Voluntary Organisations* observed that informal care is 'probably substantial in quantity: we have no doubt that a great deal more of it goes on than is commonly recognised'. At the time, policy makers, service providers and the general public, including parents themselves, were also vague about the notion of 'carers', failing to acknowledge the difference from normal family roles. Consequently, services could not have been as responsive or well-targeted as the community care situation required. By this time however, England was facing a detrimental economic situation that culminated in the 'winter of discontent' and brought a crippling halt to the welfare effort.

Conservative efforts (1979–1989)

By the end of the 1970s and beginning of the 1980s, a new discourse of disability rights emerged from the UK Disability Movement, largely led by the Union of the Physically Impaired Against Segregation (UPIAS), based on a social model of disability. They argued that it is systemic barriers, negative attitudes and exclusion by society (purposely or inadvertently), and not a person's impairment, that is disabling (Oliver, 1983). This changed the way people with disabilities were conceptualised in society, from a medical case, to a new paradigm where citizens were being disabled by society's failure to take account of and include people regardless of their individual differences.

However, while this new model undoubtedly changed the way people with disabilities were treated, at the time, as a result of the economic recession at the end of the 1970s, the issue of welfare reform was high on the agenda. The newly elected Conservative government denounced the Welfare State for creating a dependency culture with its first White Paper on public spending plans beginning with the bold statement; 'Public expenditure is at the heart of Britain's present economic difficulties' (HM Treasury, 1979). The government placed heavy blame on the welfare state for the nation's economic and moral decline. It claimed that state welfare had contributed to deindustrialisation, had created disincentives and had caused demoralisation (Clarke and Langan, 2001b). This became the guiding theme in government policy; to 'shake off the shackles of socialism', and to encourage people to take responsibility for their own lives (p. 52).

An era of retrenchment from 1979 until the early 1990s challenged the principle of a universal system of welfare. An expanded private market and role for the voluntary sector and the greater involvement of families and communities in the care of dependent groups filled this gap. A mixed approach to welfare (or 'welfare pluralism') provided the major framework for policy-making (Ruggie, 1996). The Conservative's main aim of welfare pluralism was to break up the state's monopoly of welfare provision, creating enhanced roles for private and voluntary sector alternatives and thereby allowing welfare 'consumers' to exercise greater choice among different welfare providers. The social democratic model based on universal principles was substantially eroded and a neo-conservative model based on selectivity and residualism became a more dominant model, based on principles of individualism, privatisation and marketisation of welfare provision (Esping-Andersen, 2000).

During this period, the cost savings of deinstitutionalisation were often being achieved, however, not because care in the community was in itself a cheaper option but because many of the services needed to support those with intellectual disability adequately in the community were not being fully developed (Quin and Redmond, 2005). Goodwin (1997) argued that the government's less than comprehensive community plans added to the suspicion that they were more interested in fiscal rectitude than comprehensive community care (Anderson, 1990). The withdrawal of government expenditure on human services was largely legitimised as a result of the potential for economic savings by the state during the recession.

As a result of reduced funding for public social services, community care services relied increasingly on the unpaid help of families (Clarke and Langan, 2001b). The discourse of care shifted towards 'freeing' the family from the state, enabling the restoration of responsibilities to the family which had been appropriated by the state and thereby reinforced parental responsibility and authority. Privatisation in social services in reality then involved the transfer of responsibility to the *private* realm of the family. This increased expectation of the family role was reflected in the introduction of the Invalid Care Allowance (established under the *Social Security Act* (1975)). It was given to those caring for those who received the middle or highest rate care component of 'Disability Living Allowance', or certain rates of 'Constant Attendance Allowance'.

Given the prevailing gender distribution of care within families, this implicit transfer of care responsibilities meant an increase in female domestic labour – the 'labour of love' which is embodied in women's family obligations (Finch, 1989). These gender assumptions were in some cases, an explicit part of the Conservatives agenda. In a speech to the 1977 Conservative Party Conference, a future Secretary of State for Social Services, Patrick Jenkin, expressed this view of primary care in a definitive way:

> Quite frankly, I don't think that mothers have the same right to work as fathers do. If the good Lord had intended us to have equal rights to go out to work, he wouldn't have created men and women. These are biological facts...We hear a lot today about social work – perhaps the most important social work is motherhood (quoted in Clarke, Cochrane, and Smart, 1987: 140).

While this gender stereotype remained within the Conservative government's official ethos for some time after this, the discourse of 'family carer' finally came into government discourse in the 1980s. In 1980, the government asked the National Institute of Social Work (NISW) to carry out a review of the social services system. NISW set up an independent committee, chaired by Peter Barclay. The Barclay report in 1982 made wide-ranging recommendations about the role of social workers, but more importantly made a 'discovery' of the amount of care provided by and within families at this time. This led to the work of women in providing care being dignified through the concept of 'primary carer'. Against this all other forms of care (provided by the state or other agencies) were viewed as the provision of secondary care – support for the work of primary carers (Barclay Committee, 1982).The report observed that:

> The bulk of social care in England and Wales is provided, not by the statutory or voluntary social services agencies, but by ordinary people who may be linked into informal caring networks in their communities. (Barclay Report, 1982, pp. 199–200)

Barclay placed great emphasis on the significance of these informal caring networks, and on the need for formal social services to work closely with them, not in isolation. Social workers were encouraged to find ways of developing partnerships with people with disabilities, informal carers, statutory services and voluntary agencies and suggested a shift from a counselling orientation to one concerned with social care planning. Community social work formed an important part in this strategic shift (Bulmer, 1987). The Barclay committee saw itself as repeating what the Seehohm committee had advocated in the late 1960s, with the difference that, in the early 1980s, the Conservative government's emphasis on welfare pluralism ironically presented favourable circumstances for a shift in this direction.

In the mid-1980s, a number of reports were highly critical of government failure to develop any coherent community care policies, thus adopting a similar line to the *Barclay Report* (1982). In 1986, an independent group called the *Audit Commission* published a report: *Making a Reality of Community Care* which was important in the developments of the community care changes which were to take place (Powell, 2001). Firstly the report placed a new emphasis on managerialism, market values and increased involvement of the voluntary sector. Secondly, it identified a number of key problems with community care practice, such as the 'perverse financial incentives' which supported the development of private institutional care at the expense of community care, through income support. They also identified a lack of incentives for local authorities to promote community care options; the lack of clear financial arrangements to facilitate the re-settlement in the community of long-stay residential patients (Powell, 2001).

By this time, the Carers' National Association constituted a formidable pressure group and forced Thatcher's government to respond to the *Audit Commission* (Lewis 1999). They took action by appointing Sir Roy Griffiths to write a report on community care policy. In drafting his report, he looked at ways that resources could be used 'as a contribution to more effective community care' (Department of Health and Social Security, 1988). When SSDs were formed in 1971, the intention was to co-ordinate their activities as far as possible with health services. The *Griffiths Report* (1988), proposed a different kind of arrangement; rather than depending on co-ordination and integration of services, there should be one service with clearly defined responsibility, which would by commissioned from others. This function, in the case of community care, would be performed by SSDs. Each budget would be redirected to come under the SSDs control. In principle, the SSDs would purchase the care services from a range of providers. The departments were to develop a range of provision based on these contracts. Care managers were to be responsible for allocating resources and setting priorities; practitioners would assess individual cases and guide the selection for each person.

The Griffiths Report identified three key objectives for a new community care structure, which reflected the intensification towards consumerism in the discourse of community care: (1) a focus upon the individual user and carer – meeting need, improving choice, promoting self-determination; (2) promotion of noninstitutional support services – to be delivered in the domestic environment and community settings; (3) and effective targeting of resources – to ensure those most in need received services and to avoid inefficiency and waste of resources (Powell, 2001). The report highlighted the failure of community care policies to clarify the responsibilities of social services, health, housing, voluntary and private sectors within the field of community care. In addition, Griffiths recommended that the role of local authorities should change:

> Care and support can be provided from a variety of sources. There is value in a multiplicity of provision, not least from the consumer's point of view, because of the widening choice, flexibility, innovation and competition it should stimulate… it is vital that social services authorities should see themselves as arrangers and purchasers of care services – not as monopolistic providers (Griffiths, 1988: para. 3.4).

Health professionals and independent residential care services were less enthused about some of the Report's recommendations, with health professionals losing dominance, and owners of institutions viewing the report as hostile to residential care. The Treasury was also reluctant to ring-fence funding for community care. However, the *1989 White Paper, Caring for People* that emerged the following year took on board most of the Griffiths' recommendations, although there was no implementation of any ring-fenced funding or Minister for Community Care (Milligan, 2001). The White Paper however confirmed that the government agreed with this approach and adjured public funding agencies to develop an increasingly contractual relationship with the private sector and with voluntary organisations. By now, after being in office for a third time, Margaret Thatcher extended the internal market into the NHS, with hospital trusts and GP fundholding. This meant the establishment of 'quasi-markets', with competition between providers to supply services to separate purchasers. Initially, general practitioners were the fundholders. This saw a purchaser-provider split where purchasers, acting on behalf of service users, were able to buy services from the provider whose services best met a particular need (Douglas and Philpot, 1998). The aim was to construct a more efficient and 'business-like' model of procuring services. Poor relations prevailed for some time between the medical profession and the government, however, after some time the British Medical Association saw benefits in both hospital trusts and fundholding and GP's were keen to take advantage of the incentives by the new contract.

Commissioning has since remained a core part of the English community care structure. Some local authorities no longer provide any residential care services, purely acting as purchasers or commissioners. Others, either for political or geographical reasons, or because their own provision is the best available, have retained some direct provision like home care services, day centres and residential homes (Douglas and Philpot, 1998). The guidance that followed gave 'case managers' the responsibility of commissioning services on behalf of their clients but within a predefined overall budget (Drake, 1999: 59). It thus became an effective method of decentralisation from central state to local authorities. In terms of how this was monitored, the Social Services Inspectorate (SSI) became responsible for the registration and inspection of local authority social services.

The contract culture led to a renewed role for the voluntary sector in community care. Thatcher described volunteers as 'the heart of all our social welfare provision' (Drake, 1999: 73). Hence voluntary bodies began to represent additional 'agencies' to be drawn upon, offering a cheaper alternative to local authority services. On one hand, many voluntary agencies were unwilling to enter into new partnerships with the public sector, and reluctant to take on the task of filling gaps in the network of service provision and become subject to scrutiny by state agencies (Clarke and Langan, 2001b). For these organisations, the privatisation of the social services and the emergence of a contract culture threatened the nature, if not the very existence, of volunteering (Clarke and Langan, 2001b). On the other hand, where voluntary alternatives were well established, the new model posed few problems. In these cases, the contract culture promised the twin attractions of resources and security. Furthermore, some larger voluntary organisations, such as Mencap identified themselves in national debate as a permanent and indispensable part of the welfare scene in England and increasingly claimed the right to help determine the future of welfare provision by participating in its planning.

However, the spread of voluntary alternatives was by no means complete, either in terms of the range of services or geographically. As a result of the organic nature of the voluntary sector, the number of service providers increased, the act of coordination became ever more complex; as regulations were increasingly formalised, and administration lost its flexibility. According to Baxter et al. (1990), the increased emphasis at this time on voluntary organisations led to increased geographical variation and uneven spread, particularly in class and ethnic terms.

Major's Community Care Act (1990–1996)

In 1990 John Major replaced Margaret Thatcher as the Conservative Prime Minister. Health Minister William Waldegrave indicated his concern to avoid falling into the two extreme claims of on the one hand, 'It's all up to individuals', and on the other, 'It's all up to Government' (Department of Health, 1991: v). He announced arrangements for providing funds for voluntary organisations, recognising that they could play a significant part through 'self-help', 'bringing people together to share common problems'. This was perhaps the start of an early 'third way' paradigm which the later New Labour government capitalised on.

At the start of Major's term, according to the 1991 Census (Home Office, 1991), 89 per cent of adults with learning difficulties lived in the community, supported by members of their families. Family care was becoming more noticed, perhaps as a result of the policy reports over the previous few years. As one saw, prior to this, community care was characterised by a model that tended to treat carers as resources and to assume that the social care system need only intervene when informal support was unavailable (Twigg and Atkin, 1994).

The pace of legislation in health and social services began to quicken in the early 1990s, with the *Disability Living Allowance and Disability Working Allowance Act* (1991) and the *National Health Service and Community Care Act* (1990; 1993 when fully implemented). The first Act introduced the 'disability living allowance' (DLA) (and the 'disability working allowance' (DWA) which was since discontinued) which was a tax-free benefit for adults who needed help with personal care or had walking difficulties from a disability. The second Act assigned responsibility for assessing needs, putting together packages of care and funding to meet those needs to local authorities social services departments responsible for organising and funding support and care in the community. The passage of this Act can be considered as a 'defining moment' in the acceptance of care within communities as the preferred way of meeting the needs of disabled people (Barnes, 1997). It meant social workers would have the dual (and somewhat conflicting) role of advocating for people and deciding their eligibility to funding and support in the community. While the government saw this as a progressive step, a common complaint from carers was how much time social services departments spent making sure they did not go 'over budget' and how little time and effort went into 'doing proper social work' (Rummery et al., 1999). However, although the *NHS and Community Care Act* (1990) set out a clear framework for the assessment and planning of community care needs, it said little about who would be eligible for direct care services, so old legislation going back to the *National Assistance Act* (1948) still applied (Douglas and Philpot, 1998).

It was at this time however, after three election victories, that the Conservatives seriously began to extend market forces in those areas of welfare which previously had stronger public and professional support (Clarke and Langan, 2001b). This cleared the way for private sector and voluntary organisations to bid for contracts to supply services that had previously fallen within the mainstream of state responsibility. The result was that social services also underwent a purchaser/provider split. Between 1993 and 1998, 85 per cent of each local authority's government grant for new community care services had to be spent in the independent sector. As a result, the independent social care sector grew fast, like local authority social services departments did in the 1970s when they were first set up. Examples include the 'Carewatch' franchise, which became a healthcare recruitment business for people to work as care assistants and support staff (Carewatch, 2004). Many smaller suppliers began to be swallowed up and squeezed out by consortia who were rapidly diversifying into different types of provision, like any other expanding business.

Since the early 1990s, virtually every social services department in England was organised into specialist teams. Generic teams of the 1970s and 1980s who dealt with every referral were re-organised. By the late 1990s the only truly generic social services staff left were emergency duty staff, who covered every service outside normal working hours, and social workers in remote parts of the UK (Douglas and

Philpot, 1998). As a result of these changes, community care services to adults now amounts to three-quarters of all UK social services. Their sheer scale and scope make it hard to talk about them as a whole. The most popular service is home care, in which home helps visit people to perform vital domestic work and personal care tasks such as dressing someone (Douglas and Philpot, 1998).

Social services since 1990–91 have been funded through the Revenue Support Grant which is paid annually in a single block grant to each local authority to run all its services. Government indicates to local authorities what it thinks it should spend on each service, in the form of a Standard Spending Assessment (SSA) (UK Parliament, 1996). For social services, there has been an overall SSA, and within that a children's services SSA, an elderly services SSA, and an 'other' SSA which covers disability services. Two problems have emerged in relation to the SSAs. The first has been the underlying methodology for calculating SSAs has been repeatedly questioned. SSAs are calculated using a range of general population data. They are prone to miss key local trends and variations that do not necessarily show up in broad demographic profiles. At worst, the SSA is a virtual budget. Some social services departments spend 50 per cent above it, others up to 40 per cent below (Douglas and Philpot, 1998).

The second problem was that overall sums of money were inadequate and long-term funding shortfalls have remained a serious problem. As government expenditure tightened, local authorities have increasingly found themselves facing the option of either 'robbing Peter to pay Paul', or attempting to generate income through the introduction/expansion of charging policies for services (Milligan, 2001). In relation to this problem, community care changes in 1993 effectively capped spiralling public spending on residential services, by consolidating and capping budgets and transferring responsibility for managing these integrated capped budgets to local authority social services departments. Local authorities have been expected to raise as much of their budget as possible through charging disabled people for a proportion of the cost of their care packages (Douglas and Philpot, 1998). This expenditure restraint which underpinned the rhetoric of increased choice and user responsiveness has been described as being a 'deep normative core' of government policy (Lewis and Glennerster 1996).

By the mid-1990s, family carers also became more vociferous as a lobby group. Campaigning became more visible for the rights of carers, in particular from the Carers National Association (CNA), who campaigned to raise awareness of the vital role played by carers and their need for support. Given the increasing focus on 'carers' as a new constituency, the *Carers (Recognition and Services) Act* (1995), known as the *Carers Act* was passed (and implemented on April 1st 1996). Under the Act, the term 'carer' was legally recognised, along with the value and importance of the work that they do. More importantly, this gave the local authority the duty to carry out an assessment under section 47(1)(a) of the *National Health Service and Community Care Act* (1990) of the needs of the carer as well as care-recipient. Carers could request the local authority, before they make their decision as to whether the needs of the disabled individual call for the provision of any services, to carry out an assessment of the carers ability to provide and to continue to provide care for the person needing care. Prior to this, community care assessments tended to take for granted the existence of carers, and until this time, carers had no legal rights of their own. Local authorities were therefore expected to offer assessments to carers at the time or anytime after these formal assessment procedures took place. The conclusion of each assessment is set out in a care plan, which is then put into practice by a care manager. Care managers update and monitor care plans, sometimes along with 'provider co-ordinators' who work out the fine detail of daily care programmes (Douglas and Philpot, 1998). Care management is carried out by social workers or other district nurses.

The rate of legislation also continued to gather pace for disabled people during this period, as a result of the increased pressure from the disability movement. The *Disability Discrimination Act* (1995) was hugely important for signalling the headway made by supporters of the social model of disability and indicated that legislators were prepared to accept that the lives of disabled people might be affected by the social and physical environment as well as by cognitive or physiological impairments. People with physical disabilities were also at the forefront of the successful campaign to allow 'direct payments'. Until the *Community Care (Direct Payments) Act* (1996) local authorities were not permitted by law to make direct payments to users of services so that they could themselves purchase services (Douglas and Philpot, 1998). The Act also codified a growing consensus among policy makers and service providers that the distinction between those capable and those not capable of living an ordinary life within the community needed to be questioned. According to Barnes (1997) it was within the health service that the idea of community care was newly introduced to make many service providers change their assumption that the needs of those with a disability should be met within a hospital environment. However, there were many teething problems with this legislation. Firstly, some payments were very small and secondly, the law was permissive, not mandatory. In other words, local authorities were allowed to offer direct payments, but were not compelled to.

In terms of social services, at the end of Major's term in office, a new programme of 'joint reviews' of local authority social services departments was undertaken by the SSI (1996) in conjunction with the public spending watchdog, the Audit Commission, in which each local authority's overall performance on social services was reviewed. The general findings were that while some department's exceled in some functions or in providing some specialist services, very few were found to excel in everything they did (Douglas and Philpot, 1998).

New Labour: Caring about the Carers (1997–Present)

The Labour Party won the 1997 General Election by a landslide, after 18 years in opposition. The British general election in 1997 constituted a rejection of new-conservatism, however New Labour were also wary of causing 'reorganisation fatigue' (Paton, 1999: 57). The change of government introduced ideas and new policies related to social inclusion and a restructuring of local government services. The New Labour government, when elected, emphasised its break with 'Old Labour' and its distinctiveness from Thatcherism, advocating what it described as a 'third way'. In its welfare reform Green Paper this is explicit:

> The welfare state now faces a choice of futures. A privatised future, with the welfare state becoming a residual safety net for the poorest and most marginalised; the status quo, but with more generous benefits; or the Government's third way – promoting opportunity instead of dependence, with a welfare state providing for the mass of the people, but in new ways to fit the modern world. (Department of Social Services, 1998)

In practice, it is still hard to establish precisely what New Labour actually meant by its 'third way'. As far as public spending was concerned, it made great efforts to shed the 'tax and spend' image of Old Labour, and embraced tight public spending limits from 1997–99, as set by its Conservative predecessor (Hills, 1998). In this sense its policies marked little change from before. However it managed to produce significant extra spending in popular areas without the kind of politically damaging tax increases which might have been expected as the way of paying for them under Old Labour.

In its first year, the government established the *Royal Commission on Long Term Care*. Its terms of reference were 'to examine the short and long term options for a *sustainable* system of funding of Long Term Care, both in their own homes and other settings.' The Government also made clear attempts at putting carers on the map with their White Paper *Modernising Social Services* (1998). It noted that the care system had not adequately recognised the enormous contribution that informal carers make to maintain the independence of people with care needs (Department of Social Services, 1998). According to the Office for National Statistics, in 1998, Britain had an estimated 5.7 million family carers, with one in six households – 17 per cent – containing a carer (cited in UK Government, 1999). Of these carers, 58 per cent were women; 60 per cent said they were looking after someone with a physical disability, with a further 15 per cent looking after someone with both a mental and a physical disability. 1.7 million devoted at least 20 hours a week to caring, and of those, 855,000 cared for 50 hours a week or more. People who share a household with their care recipient tend to spend more of their time caring – 38 per cent spending at least 50 hours a week. In terms of their economic status, 49 per cent of carers were working, either full or part-time. This finally gave a national picture of the extent and characteristics of caregiving; and re-framed the discourse of 'carers' as a constituency distinct from regular parents.

In terms of disability policy, the Labour Party manifesto for the 1997 general election promised disabled people a Disability Rights Commission to provide support for the *Disability Discrimination Act* (1995) comparable to those bodies safeguarding the rights of women and ethnic minorities. However, the *Disability Discrimination Act* (1995) has so far proved to be disappointingly weak. In a test case in 1997, the Law Lords decided that Gloucestershire Social Services was not compelled to provide services if it could not command the necessary resources (Drewett, 1999). The government's own compliance cost assessment estimated that implementing the comprehensive civil rights legislation envisaged in the Rights Bill, might require as much as £17 billion in (non-recurring) capital expenditure and a further £1 billion per annum in revenue costs (Drake, 1999). However, the *Rights Now* organisation argued that the assessment contained serious flaws and maintained that the cost of implementing the Bill could be some £12 billion less. The group also calculated substantial cost benefits (between £2.25 and £5 billion per annum) accruing where disabled people found work and ended their dependence on social security payments. Indeed as we shall see, the *Americans with Disabilities Act* led to minimal extra costs on American business and actually resulted in the opening up of several new market opportunities for those providing goods and services to disabled consumers (Berven and Blanck, 1998).

In attempting to construct a new landscape of care, New Labour drew up plans for bringing NHS and local authority social services together to overcome the politically unacceptable levels of geographic variation in the level and quality of community health services across England (Hills, 1998). As a result, New Labour set up National Service Frameworks (NSF) to overcome much of the variation. Each NSF was developed with the assistance of an External Reference Group (ERG) which brings together health professionals, service users and carers, health service managers, partner agencies, and other advocates. The NSF's are now responsible for: setting national standards and identify key interventions for a defined service or care group; putting in place strategies to support implementation; establishing ways to ensure progress within an agreed time scale; and raising quality and decreasing variations in service (Department of Health, 2005a).

In their NHS Plan, New Labour asserted that their efforts to modernise services 'all too often founder on the fault lines in the NHS which are a hangover from the world of 1948' (Department of Health, 2000). New Labour also attributed these regional variations which developed gradually but steadily after 1966 as a result of the Conservative's NHS internal market. Their White Paper *The New NHS: Modern, Dependable* was published in December 1997, some seven months after the government took office, and focused on a major decentralisation of the health and social care system. It proposed the closer integration of health and social care services at all levels, from the integration of health and social services policy within the Department of Health at the top, to new statutory duties on all NHS organisations to work in partnership with local authorities (Rummery and Glendinning, 2000).

With the *NHS Act* (1999), New Labour set up Primary Care Groups (PCGs) within the Health Authority regions. These were new local, devolved organisational frameworks which emphasised horizontal coordination and integration of services within a locality. The proposals in the Act were aimed at unifying virtually all health services funding streams and devolving responsibility for managing the budget to local PCGs (Our Healthier Nation, 2004). These all became free-standing Primary Care Trusts (PCTs) over time. Their prime role has since been in developing primary care, commissioning residential services for people with disabilities and improving local health. By 2005, there were 481 PCTs across the country with responsibility for approximately 75 per cent of the NHS budget (Department of Health, 2005b). This decentralisation of financial decision making through budget holding was seen as an important instrument for making more cost-effective use of scarce resources.

Meanwhile 28 new strategic Health Authorities were created in 2002 to manage the NHS locally and to act as a key link between the Department of Health and the PCTs. They are responsible for developing plans for improving health services in their local area, making sure local health services are of a high quality and are performing well, and increasing the capacity of local health services so they can provide more services (NHS, 2005). In addition, a small number of Care Trusts were set up around the country to work in both health and social care. They have been established in a discretionary manner when the NHS and Local Authorities agree to work closely together, usually where it is felt that a closer relationship between health and social care is needed or would benefit local care services, though more will be set up in the future. They may carry out a range of services, including social care, mental health services or primary care services (NHS, 2005).

As well as the *NHS Act* (1999), that same year three different policy reports for carers were published to assess where services were at and how to address carers' issues in future, thus signalling the new-found commitment to carers as a separate constituency: *A National Strategy 'Caring for Carers'*; the *Royal Commission's Report on Long Term Care*; and a *Note of Dissent by Members of The Royal Commission*. The first of these, the National Strategy (UK Government, 1999), recommended the provision of three elements for carers: *information*, *support* and *care* and a 'joined up government' approach to overcome geographical issues in governance. The section on information stressed the importance of involving carers in decision-making. Carers should be informed and consulted about professional decision-making concerning those they care for. Secondly, carers' views should be taken into account when planning community care services. Since then, the development and writing of the *Valuing People* (2001) strategy was a major attempt by Government to include the voices of carers and individuals with intellectual disabilities (Rolph et al., 2006). The section on support referred to a range of provision, including health, social services, transport and in particular, housing. Finally, the section on 'care' was to provide short-term breaks from caring. The strategy proposed a new special grant providing £140m for England over a three-year period to enable carers to take short-term breaks from caring. This approach differed from the Royal Commission's policy statement, in that carers were focused upon directly. This recognition of the need for regular breaks as opposed to 'respite', with its connotations of relief from suffering, was important. However, it was recognised that without adequate funds, the good practice guidelines were of limited value (Lloyd, 2000).

The Royal Commission's report contained only a short section on carers. Nevertheless, two of its 24 recommendations concerned carers; the first proposing better services should be offered to those people who currently have a carer; and the second, that the government should consider a national carers' support package. Pickard (2001) uses the term 'carer blind' to illustrate the intention of the report. Services which are carer blind mean that the existence of a carer will not lead to the failure to offer services. In this instance, the focus of intervention was not the carer but the care recipient, thus indirectly providing support for the carer. The Commission estimated that to provide services on a carer-blind basis, would cost £290m and that, in addition to the money provided under the National Carers' Strategy, a further £220m was needed.

In addition to this, a '*Note of Dissent*' from the Royal Commission was written by two of its members to set out their points of disagreement to their report. They argued that more emphasis needed to be placed on help for informal carers than was given in the report. This reflects the crosscutting discourses which were beginning to emerge in the care literature, from the 'disability rights' perspective and the feminist care perspective. Those writing from the disability rights perspective have argued that policy should focus on endorsing independence for the disabled person, thus underwriting the dependence on carers. On the other hand, feminist writers have argued that as long as women continue to be the primary carers in the home, the emotional component of care, and care work more generally, will remain undervalued (see Milligan and Power, 2009).

What seems clear is that each approach contained in the policy documents seems on its own to be insufficient. A comprehensive joined-up approach should encompass both support for carers *and* support for those they care for, or at least a common vision so that one 'constituency' is not emancipated at the expense of the other.

Since these three reports, there has been continued Government interest in improving support to carers. However, in the years following the introduction of the 1995 Carers Act, carer assessments were few and if carried out at all, were part of the person with the disabilities' assessment rather than separately. Carer assessments were not an established feature of practice. Despite this right being subsequently extended by the *Carers and Disabled Children Act* (2000), according to Seddon et al. (2007), practitioners voiced concerns about completing carer assessments and they were careful to avoid raising carer expectations. Practitioners maintained that separate carer assessments were time-consuming and administratively burdensome and that they had to identify support needs which services were unable to address.

The commitment by the UK Government to supporting carers has been described as one of the most striking developments in social policy (Moriarty and Webb, 2000). However, it must be asked to what extent has the changes stemming from all the recent carer policy affected the landscape of care at the local scale?

Firstly, according to the Commission for Social Care Inspection report (previously the Social Service Inspectorate) (November 2004), performance varies between councils, in terms of their role in affecting access to services, for many of the indicators but overall the variation reduced for the fifth successive year since 2000. The strongest performance was evident in the North East, East Midlands and Yorkshire and Humber regions. The North East and London, followed by the Eastern region, saw the strongest rate of improvement over the last year of the evaluation. In population terms, social care performance improved for councils containing 14 per cent of the population. For councils serving nearly 80 per cent of the population, performance ratings stayed the same, and for councils serving 8 per cent of the population, performance deteriorated.

Secondly, in terms of the regional variation between local health authorities, according to Rummery and Glendinning (2002), a considerable risk of fragmentation and variation remains *between* the PCTs within any one area. The Health Authority's *Health Investment Plan* is the key mechanism for providing overall strategic coherence between the different PCTs within its boundaries. However it is unclear how effective this will be to bring about cohesion. Furthermore, the legislation has meant that at the board level of the PCTs, there is a conflation of professional power, which was previously held by social workers, GPs and nurses, with managerial power over resources, previously held by health authorities. Often there is conflicting demands of managerial gate-keeping and professional ethics (Rummery and Glendinning, 2000).

Thirdly, in terms of local authority social service departments, since the community care changes in the late 1980s/90s, and events since, many local authorities have devolved their budgets down to front-line teams and agencies, so that local managers can use their part of the budget flexibly to support people with the greatest needs in their part of the service. Devolution can eliminate the inherent delays and administration costs in constantly referring expenditure proposals up the hierarchy, as long as local managers know the rules about what can and cannot be spent, and as long as they are supplied with an accurate financial monitoring system (Douglas and Philpot, 1998). However, as a result of the devolution, carers have to access an assessment in order to access services. Social workers were therefore given the opportunity to ration both services and resources in their assessments. The legislation therefore shifted the managerial responsibility to ration access to scarce resources from managers to professionals without placing those professionals under any substantive obligations to be accountable to local citizens or involve them in any significant way in the process (Seddon et al., 2007).

Finally, as a result of these changes, there are clear examples of rationing of health and social services on the ground. Arksey (2002) has classified the different sorts of rationing that exist in the administration and allocation of services into seven types: by denial, by selection, by deterrence, by dilution, by delay, by substitution and by charges. This has also contributed to a phenomenon of carers imposing rationing on themselves. Many carers now impose their own limits on the amount of help they ask for, while some feel guilty for accepting any outside help (Arskey, 2002).

Despite the role of the 1995 *Carers Act* in significantly raising awareness of carers' issues, it made little difference to the numbers of carers receiving assessments. The voluntary sector recognises this as a huge issue and continue to address it through their own information services. For example, a group called *Signposts* offers an unofficial assessment service for carers in order to make the process easier (Signposts, 2003). Family carers of people with learning disabilities over the age of 18 in particular find themselves in a very different situation from that of other carers because they are not suddenly struggling with a new role, but have built up their coping strategies over their relative's lifetime. Thus many simply try and cope without having an assessment (Robinson and Williams, 2002).

As a result, the percentages of carer assessments and reviews were still low across England (59 per cent and 20 per cent respectively) (Commission for Social Care Inspection, 2004). Within the Eastern region, according to the *Regional Monitoring Report* (2002), performance on Carer's assessments is average, but with very large regional variations between 27 per cent and 79 per cent. Clearly, therefore, regional disparities are evident across England. The individual aspects of England's local authority social services departments present a picture of quite complex and variegated geographical differentiation across local areas, however at the broader spatial scale, distinct regional patterns are less clear. Although the local authorities are closely monitored, the individual nature of their remit will continue to make regions vulnerable to geographical differences in care services.

Evidence already exists that carers are going to continue being at the forefront of policy attention for the foreseeable future in England with the recent *Carers (Equal Opportunities) Act* (2004), which was drafted by an MP and long-advocate of carers, Dr Hywel Francis. Dr Francis had originally envisaged the legislation to have a wide scope around health, employment and life-long learning for carers. However the Act merely mandates a duty on adult services to *inform* carers of their right to an assessment and to ensure a carer's wishes for employment, learning or training opportunities and leisure are *considered* as part of the carer's assessment. As a result, according to Seddon et al. (2007), there has been a considerable and enduring gap between policy and practice over the ten years since the 1995 *Carers (Recognition and Services) Act*. In their study of the assessment of carer need over time, they identify practitioners' reluctance to offer separate carer assessments, as well as confusion relating to the interpretation of eligibility criteria and the limited contribution of health service staff.

Disability rights were also extended in 2005 with the *Disability Discrimination Act 2005*, which makes substantial amendments to the *Disability Discrimination Act 1995*. The DDA represents a new approach. It focuses on institutional change rather than adjustments for individuals. It places a duty on all public bodies to promote disability equality. For example, it imposes a specific duty on key public bodies, such as higher education institutions, to produce a disability equality scheme (DES). The DES must consider the impact of all current and proposed institutional activities (e.g. plans, policies, procedures) on disabled people and provide an explanation of how impact will be assessed. It also must show how progress on disability equality will be measured and how they will monitor and evaluate their action plans.

In the same year as the DDA was enacted, the Government also embarked on a major reversal of earlier decentralisation policy, in order to reduce the amount of local Primary Care Trusts. It announced that the number of Strategic Health Authorities and Primary Care Trusts would be reduced, the latter by about 50 per cent. The result is that, as of 1 October 2006, there are 10 Strategic Health Authorities (SHAs) (reduced from 28) and 152 PCTs (reduced from 481) in England, with an average population of just under 330,000 per trust. Only the London PCTs have remained with their former boundaries. After these changes, about 70 per cent of PCTs are co-terminous with local authorities having social service responsibilities, which it is hoped will facilitate joint planning. The fewer, more strategic organisations will deliver stronger commissioning functions. It is also hoped that the mergers will release about £259m in annual savings for the NHS (NHS, 2010).

Finally, in terms of adult social care, by the mid-2000s, there has been a stronger policy emphasis on personalisation. This emerged largely from the work of In Control who strategically developed a Resource Allocation System for local authorities to use a model of allocating individualised funding. Many disability groups called for direct payments to give adults with intellectual disabilities and their families more choice in designing their own support system. Person centred planning, advocacy and direct payments were at the heart of the original Valuing People (2001). The subsequent Valuing People Now report (2009) also recommended that more people with learning disabilities should be able to commission their own services to live independently and have real choice about the way they live their lives. However, in the national consultation for the report (Hatton et al., 2009), it was argued by a significant amount of family carers that direct payments simply added more workloads to carers by having to manage budgets and design care support arrangements for their children. This threat has also been highlighted by Glendining (2009) and Glendinning et al. (2009) in their research into the impacts and outcomes for carers of individual budgets. England therefore appears to be at a crossroads in how they are going to arrange their adult social care system in the future. However, given the limitations of traditional models of support which often restrict the choices of adults with intellectual disabilities and a newly elected coalition government (on 6 May 2010), England will likely follow the US' lead and offer policy options which encourage individuals and their families to lead their own support plans.

Conclusion

The history of 'care' in England takes us into a realm of shifting ideas and conceptions of disability and the family itself. In the area of legislation and policy, carers have become recognised as both a source of care and in need of care themselves. In a period of over a hundred years, the notion of what constitutes 'Care' has changed a great deal from containment and exclusion to care in the community. As well as focusing on the policy climate, this chapter has examined the changing discourses through time, from the 'deserving' and 'non-deserving' disabled distinction in the 1940s and 1950s, to normalisation and social role valorisation in the 1960s and 1970s, and later to the recognition of family carers in mainstream society as a group in need of support in the 1990s and early 2000s.

Grand statements about carers' interests predominating over those of professionals will ring hollow unless those interests are given practical effect in the way services are shaped and provided. While overcoming the marginalisation of carers requires a politics of cultural recognition and a politics of political representation, it also requires a politics of economic redistribution. All three are essential for advancing toward full citizenship for all members of society (Prince, 2009). The funding framework for community care, however, has proven problematic. Budgets are allocated to local authorities from central government. Most monies, however are not specifically earmarked for care services – rather they have to be argued for at a local level from general rate support money (Milligan, 1999).

In terms of the changing site of care towards the home, seeing the spatial configuration of how community care policies have worked on the ground has helped to resist the assumption of an over-simplistic notion of progress. Rather one should acknowledge that while 'improvements' have been made, in other respects the scenario is more mixed. When looked at more closely, the transition between Thatcherite conservative policies and those of New Labour has been less clear. England in more recent times has moved towards relying on the market and self responsibility in administering care support.

What is striking is that even New Labour have distanced themselves from the 1945 post-war welfare reforms and 'the pre-historic NHS structure' of the time (Department of Health, 2000). On one side, this period in English history was seen a triumphal moment – the point at which British society was transformed and a peculiarly British variety of welfare was installed. On the other side the conservatives argue that it was a low point: an excessive and excessively interfering structure which undermined British freedoms (Cochrane and Clarke, 1993).

Over the last 10 years, there has been a resurgence in addressing the lack of community-care developments throughout the 1970s and 1980s. The evidence suggests that the legislative efforts to acknowledge carers and their right to an 'assessment of need' singles out England in carer policy as quite progressive. On the other hand, resources for on-the-ground support are always being stretched. To put it in context, an ex-social worker and current lobbyist for Carers UK in Lancashire said:

> We get a lot of complaints from social services but at the end of the day, I'm a retired social-worker, so I know what the social workers are going through. They've a tremendous case-load to work through, they don't have sufficient

> funds to do it and they haven't sufficient social workers. There never will be sufficient social workers to provide a proper service – until the government provides the money. They do a good job, it's no good saying they don't. They do their job to the best of their ability, with the funds that are available. But they're just keeping the service ticking over.

While this stretching of social services shall no doubt remain a feature of England's neo-liberal welfare state, for the most part, England comparatively has quite a comprehensive landscape of care, made up of quasi-markets of non-profit and private service providers, non-means tested government benefits, and an assessment of carers' needs. However, given England's recent emphasis on consumerist approaches to choice in public services, there is a risk of placing a heavier weight on families to lead and manage their adult children's own support plans, without the necessary assistance to help them in this process.

Chapter 5
Caregiver's Policy in the United States

The welfare regime in the United States, in comparison to England, is described as representing individualism, laissez-faire, residualism and a punitive view of poverty. These issues often seem to dominate US debates on welfare: examples are the introduction of 'workfare', the exclusion of long-term benefit dependents, and the criticism of the 'underclass' (Spicker, 2003). According to Keigher and Stone (1994), this unwillingness to fill the gap in the welfare system originates in the larger context of American democratic customs and interest-based capitalism. Cultural traditions emphasising individual freedom, trust in family, and fear of big government remain embedded in public policy. Some US commentators have even argued that guaranteeing health care should neither be a right nor a responsibility of government:

> It is not; no one has a "right" to health care. Second, assuming that health care were a legitimate responsibility of the government and the federal government ought to "do something" about the so-called health care "crisis" [...]. The problem – if there is one – with the American health care system is that it is overinsured; we need less insurance, not more. (Mayer, 1994)

This has been a dominant and long-held debate in US health care policy. The principle of universality in terms of welfare is absent in the United States. Only Social Security begins to approach universality of coverage, however its benefits are limited to subsets of the disability population.

In practice, the US welfare state is pluralistic, in that there are significant departures from the residual model (particularly when state social welfare institutions come into play), for example state schooling and home care programmes (Spicker, 2003). Federalism has meant that many important functions are administered and legislated for by the states, including public assistance, social care and various health schemes. Long-term care policies and programmes are determined by 50 separate state governments, each with different demographics, economies and political philosophies. The American constitution specifies a certain division of responsibilities, both functional and fiscal, between units of government. One of the major explanations in the literature for the development of national health and welfare states in other countries is increasing centralisation of authority at the national level; hence the persistence of strong decentralised government in the US being cited as a significant factor for the America's lagging welfare state (Ruggie, 1996). This chapter is concerned with how family carers and their adult children with intellectual disabilities have been conceptualised and catered for in such a system, tracing the origins of its 'care' policy (see timeline in Table 5.1 overleaf), from broader federal welfare provision, to local provision across states.

The Development of Welfare and Social Services

Before independence in the US, welfare reflected English poor law quite closely. People with intellectual disabilities were generally kept at home with their families, with little or no outside support, as anyone with relatives capable of caring for them could be denied relief (Ferguson 2004). In the mid-1800s, caregivers of disabled siblings were depicted as dedicated, loving, and spiritually improved by their challenges. Being intellectually disabled did not disqualify them from work, education, social invitations, or travel. The development of early schools for people with 'mental retardation' and other disabilities in the US had its beginnings in 1848 with an experimental school in Boston.

However from the mid-19th century the learned reasoning changed to believe that parents of 'idiots' were diseased and sinful, and began to experience increasing shame and despair as the century passed (Richards, 2004). By 1877, a medical model of mental retardation that viewed people as sick and incurable had come to prominence. Likewise, the service philosophy changed to 'sheltering the deviant from society' (Evans, 1983).

From the late 19th century, industry developed rapidly and the economy tended increasingly to be characterised by industrialisation and urbanisation. A trickle-down economic philosophy was overriding and many Americans believed that private enterprise, if left alone by government, would result in unlimited prosperity (Dinsmore, 2000). Both the states and the Federal government recognised that certain risks in an increasingly industrialised economy could best be met through a *social insurance* approach to welfare, making industry responsible for the costs of compensating workers or their survivors when injured or killed in connection with the job (Social Security Online, 2003). Outside of insurance, there was no systematic method for social welfare, just individual charity groups funded by private donors (Schultz 2004). Those who advocated a larger role for government were stigmatised as radicals, communists, or traitors (Dinsmore, 2000).

This reliance on *social insurance* tended to view disabled people as 'undeserving', as a result of their inability to contribute to their own insurance. With the discovery of the principles of eugenics in the 1910s and 1920s, protection of society from the deviant became more ubiquitous and was defined in the broadest of terms, including a new concern for the protection of the gene pool (Disability Social History Project, 2003). In 1912, the American Breeders' Association produced a report regarding the best practice in cutting off defective germ plasm in the human population (Smith, 2006). 'Mentally retarded' people were therefore subjected to unnecessary institutionalisation and lifelong custody. Erving Goffman's seminal work, *Asylums* (1961) argued that this period of institutionalisation robbed patients of their individuality and writers such as Jack Tizard (1960, 1964) identified the detrimental

Table 5.1 US Disability and Care Legislation

Beginning of Eugenics.	*1907 Indiana Sterilization Act*	Indiana became the first state to enact sterilisation legislation followed closely by Washington and California.
Made distinction between 'deserving' and 'non-deserving' disabled persons.	*1918 Veterans Rehabilitation Act*	Veterans Benefits for the war disabled after World War One.
	1920 Vocational Rehabilitation Act	First of a long line of federal Acts serving the huge rate of injured. Foundation for one of the largest disability policy areas today.
Eugenics ideals became dominant.	*1924 Sterilization Act*	The Commonwealth of Virginia passed a state law that allowed for sterilisation (without consent) of individuals found to be feebleminded or insane.
	1927 U.S. Supreme Court ruling, Buck v. Bell	Ruled that the forced sterilisation of people with disabilities was not a violation of their constitutional rights.
New Deal established new role for the state.	*1935 Social Security Act*	Established two social insurance programs on a national scale to help with old age and blindness, and the risks of unemployment.
Replaced Eugenics with ideas of rehabilitation.	*1943 Barden-LaFollette Act*	Rehabilitation program for people with intellectual disabilities. To be eligible, there had to be a reasonable expectation that vocational rehabilitation may render the individual fit to engage in a remunerative occupation.
	1946 Hill-Burton Act (also known as the Hospital Survey and Construction Act)	Authorised federal grants to states for the construction of hospitals, public health centers and health facilities for rehabilitation of people with disabilities.
	1950 Social Security Act Amendments	Established a federal-state program to aid permanently and totally disabled persons.
	1954 U.S. Supreme Court ruling, Brown v. Board of Education	Affirmed the right of all citizens to an equal education.
Reinforced attention to young physically disabled over other disabilities.	*Post-World War Two*	Veterans were provided vocational rehabilitation, unemployment allowances, educational and training benefits, and job placement services.

Table 5.1 continued

	1956 Social Security Act	Set up Social Security Disability Insurance (SSDI). Benefits were provided for severely disabled workers aged 50 or older and for adult disabled children of deceased or retired workers.
	1958 Social Security Act amendments	Amended to provide benefits for dependents of disabled workers.
	1960 Social Security Act amendments	Further amended to remove the age-50 requirement for disabled-worker benefits.
Idea of rights was brought on the social agenda.	*1964 Civil Rights Act*	Outlawed discrimination on the basis of race in public accommodations and employment, as well as in federally assisted programs. Although disability or caregiving was not on the agenda, it became a model for subsequent disability rights legislation.
Acknowledged need for greater federal role in health care.	*1965 Social Security Act amendments*	Created Medicare & Medicaid providing federally subsidised health care to disabled Americans covered by the Social Security program.
First acknowledgement of intellectual disability in a more positive sense.	*1963 Mental Retardation Facilities and Community Mental Health Construction Act*	Provided funding for the formation of research and services to individuals with mental retardation and their families.
	1968 Architectural Barriers Act	Prohibited architectural barriers in all federally owned or leased buildings.
	1971 Fair Labor Standard Act Amendment	Brought people with disabilities (other than blindness) into the sheltered workshop system.
	1972 Social Security Act amendments	Created the Supplemental Security Income (SSI) means-tested program, which federalised existing State cash assistance programs. The law relieved families of the financial responsibility of caring for their adult disabled children.
	1973 Health Maintenance Act	The federal government helped to fund the growth of 'Health Maintenance Organizations' (HMOs), which are prepaid group practices to provide prepaid health plans that enrolled members and arranged for their care from a designated provider network.

Enshrined the idea of Independent Living.	*1973 Rehabilitation Act*	Under it severely disabled persons who were judged not potentially employable were made eligible to receive such services as needed so as to enable them to live independently.
Acknowledged that care could be provided at home.	*1981 established section 1915(c) of the Social Security Act*	Gave authority to waive certain provisions of Medicaid law allowing states to provide a wide range of home and community-based services for persons with disabilities of all ages in the home. These are called Medicaid Home and Community-Based Services (HCBS) Waiver Programs.
Idea of empowering & extending rights to disabled people.	*1990 Americans with Disabilities Act*	Most sweeping disability rights legislation in history. Mandated that local, state and federal governments and programs be accessible. Outlawed discrimination against disabled people in public and private sector employment. Required access to public services and transport and required access for disabled people to educational, recreational and leisure facilities.
	1993 Family and Medical Leave Act	Required employers with more than 50 workers to permit employees to take up to 12 weeks of unpaid leave to care for a family member
	1996 Personal Responsibility and Work Opportunity Reconciliation Act (PRWORA)	Changed 'Aid to Families with Dependent Children' (AFDC) to a new program called 'Temporary Assistance for Needy Families' (TANF). Carers had to qualify for Medicaid programs separately.
	1997 Balanced Budget Act (BBA)	Gave states the option of setting up Medicaid Managed Care programs without the waivers that were usually required for such programs.
Acknowledgement that the home was preferred site of care.	*1999 Olmstead vs. L.C. and E.W.*	The Supreme Court decided that individuals with disabilities must be offered services in the most integrated setting.
Changed paradigm from traditional role of family to recognising carers.	*2001 National Family Caregiver Support Program*	Minimal support to moderate-income carers, offering advice, councelling and assistance in gaining access to services.
	2003 Family Respite Care Act	Authorised funds for the development of lifespan respite programs at the state and local levels.

effects of institutionalisation on children with intellectual disabilities. Also, as a result of the eugenics movement, states carried out involuntary sterilisation. By 1926 there were 23 states that had mandatory sterilisation laws for institutionalised residents. Between 1925 and 1955, over 50,000 mandatory sterilisations occurred in the United States (Evans, 1983).

In terms of 'caring' for people with intellectual disabilities, many state governments actually required their citizenry to assist them in locating and segregating them. Physicians, teachers, and social workers, and even the general public were to report to the government all persons 'believed by them to be feeble minded' (Evans, 1983). Families who cared for their children with intellectual disabilities were stigmatised. Some statutes authorised the removal of children with disabilities from their homes, even against the parents' wishes. The state of Washington for instance made it a crime for a parent to refuse state-ordered institutionalisation. Geographically, rural locations offered the best sites for institutions to reinforce the trends of isolation, enlargement, and economisation (Metzel 2004). Once children were institutionalised, many state laws required parents to waive all custody rights. In 1927, the US Supreme Court, in *Buck v. Bell*, ruled that the forced sterilisation of people with disabilities was not a violation of their constitutional rights. The decision removed the last restraints for eugenicists; advocating that people with disabilities be prohibited from having children (Disability Social History Project, 2003). It was only much later that people with intellectual disabilities came to be included within the set of conditions that made individuals eligible for rehabilitative services.

One area where the Federal Government accepted an early responsibility for disability was in the provision of benefits and services for persons who served in the Armed Forces. This was a key step in their particular path towards later disability legislation, which focused largely on young people with physical disabilities. After World War I, the huge rate of injured young men helped in instigating the *Soldiers Rehabilitation Act* (1918). This set the pattern for a long line of federal Acts such as the *Vocational Rehabilitation Act* (1920) serving as the foundation for one of the largest disability policy areas today. These veterans' benefits at first consisted mainly of compensation for the war-disabled, widows' pensions, and land grants. Later, emphasis was placed on service pensions and domiciliary care as well as a full-scale system of hospital and medical care benefits (Social Security Online, 2003).

New Deal and World War Two (1929–1959)

The Great Depression was a watershed in American history, with depressed stock prices, a wave of bankruptcies, and deflated prices. Soon after Herbert Hoover assumed the presidency in 1929, the economy was hit with the stock market crash which began the decline. At first, Hoover believed, like most Americans, that modest tinkering with the economic system would bring the nation out of its economic crisis. He also felt that private agencies, such as the Red Cross and family service agencies, could address the needs of unemployment and poverty-stricken Americans without governmental assistance. Hoover shared Franklin Pierce's philosophy that welfare issues belonged to local governments and private philanthropy (Dinsmore, 2000).

As the Depression got worse, the nation's confidence in Hoover began to waiver. The severity of the times made Federal action towards welfare a necessity, as neither the States nor the local communities nor private charities had the financial resources to cope with the growing need among the American people. In 1932, Franklin Delano Roosevelt was elected president and he drastically changed the course of US economics and politics by introducing strong government regulation and a package of massive public works projects called the 'New Deal'. These aimed to re-employ Americans and to build a more modern infrastructure. The previous government policies of laissez-faire were replaced by increased government control and intervention. The Federal Government first made loans, then grants, to states to pay for direct relief and work relief. After that, special Federal emergency relief and public works programs were started.

Roosevelt himself was the first physically-disabled person to be elected as President of the US. The *Social Security Act* (1935) was passed establishing two social insurance programs on a national scale to help with old age and blindness, and the risks of unemployment. The choice of old age and unemployment as the risks to be covered by social insurance was a natural development, since the Depression had wiped out much of the lifetime savings of the aged and reduced opportunities for gainful employment. According to Roosevelt, this Act was the cornerstone of the New Deal (KSAH, 2002). These programs supplemented the incomes of persons who were either ineligible for Social Security or whose benefits could not provide a basic living. The intent of Federal participation was to encourage States to adopt such programs. The law established other Federal grants to enable States to extend and strengthen maternal and child health and welfare services, and these grants became the *Aid to Families with Dependent Children Program*. The Old-Age Insurance program was made a family program when benefits for dependents of retired workers and surviving dependents of deceased workers were added. These benefits became first payable in 1940 (Social Security Online, 2003).

During Roosevelt's term, people with physical and sensory disabilities were imbued with an ethos of individualistic 'striving against the odds' or 'overcoming' their disability, with Roosevelt's life in a wheelchair as the prime example. People with intellectual disabilities, however, were still often institutionalised or subjected to social control in the community. Families still found it very hard and had few choices for their child; there was no right to a free appropriate public education, very few opportunities for people with disabilities to get job training, and housing choices were limited essentially to institutions or living at home until the parents got too old. The earlier stigma from the start of the century attached to having a family member with a disability continued – people ignorantly thought that 'mental retardation' was contagious, or was an indication of poor genes in the family. One notable change however was that during the 1930s, more emphasis was placed on the study of behaviour and physiology as predispositions to intellectual disability. Jackson (1935) for instance surveyed 3,548 children with intellectual disability and reported that 281 were hypothyroid. Similarly, there were studies of the links to profound jaundice in the newborn (Diamond et al., 1932). At the same time, Doll, (1936) developed the Vineland Social Maturity Scale as a measure of adaptive behaviour, social competence, and self-help skills, from infancy to adulthood. It was used in planning for therapy and/or individualised instruction for persons with 'mental retardation'. These would begin to slowly filter into the change of discourse of intellectual disability.

Towards the end of the 1930s, it was unclear whether the social reforms of 1933 and 1934 would be maintained or dismantled. Roosevelt's second term (1937–41), although winning an even more decisive victory than in 1932, produced rising conflict and opposition as businessmen mourned the end of 'laissez-faire' and chafed under the new regulations (KSAH, 2002). Many bitterly opposed his effort in 1937 to crowd the Supreme Court with pro-New Deal justices (Chartier, 1999). Even though these changes were considered ambitious by American standards, the reforms were relatively conservative by international and today's standards (George and Taylor-Gooby, 1996). However, socialism was strongly stigmatised in the US with the labour-intensive South resistant to a truly universalistic social security system. Also, African Americans were still living under oppressive laws in the South, and faced mass unrest and residential segregation in the North. This stalled welfare further as developers did not want to apply any welfare initiatives for this population. Ultimately the middle class was not wooed from the market to the state and the majority felt the market could better satisfy its needs (Dinsmore, 2000).

On the other hand, policies and ideas that had been taboo or restricted to a few reformers were now both acceptable and operational. In a certain sense, it is fair to say the New Deal merely introduced types of social and economic reform familiar to many Europeans for more than a generation. Federal authorities could now develop national programs with greater speed and efficiency. Once the new policies were in place, there was no turning back to the restrictive welfare traditions of the 19th century; Americans had seen that the new policies, though imperfect, were preferable to the traditional approaches, which now seemed mean-minded and anachronistic (Dinsmore, 2000).

In any case, the US's joining of World War Two in 1941 caused an enormous growth in the economy as war goods and services were once again in great demand (Chartier, 1999). The *Social Security Act* (1935) brought about the start of income replacement benefits. Further developments took place in managed care just before the war in 1938, which contributed greatly towards the US healthcare system (Tufts Managed Care Institute, 1998). 'Managed care' – a system of providers where the types of care and services are overseen inside of a network – became a popular system for paying, delivering and coordinating health services. It since became the model the US has developed as their own breed of a national health service, although its role in disability support has remained contentious, as discussed later.

Staunch opposition existed to any prepaid cooperative plans however, in particular by the American Medical Association (AMA). They were opposed to any form of lay control (i.e., non-physician control) over medical professionals or anything resembling the 'corporate practice' of medicine. Later they changed their position from official sponsorship of reprisals against prepaid group practice to watchful coexistence (Tufts Managed Care Institute, 1998).

For people with intellectual disabilities during the 1940s, the rehabilitation programme was expanded with the passage of the *Barden-LaFollette Act* (1943) to include this group. However, to be eligible, individuals had to experience (i) the presence of a physical or mental disability, (ii) the existence of a substantial handicap to employment caused by the limitations present; and (iii) a reasonable expectation that vocational rehabilitation may render the individual fit to engage in a remunerative occupation. It therefore was viewed as an investment in human capital, intended to be paid off through reduced social support spending (Percy, 2001: 242). However, doctors and mental health professionals continued to argue that the only way to 'protect' the family, especially non-disabled siblings, was to institutionalise the disabled child at a very young age. According to Brockley (2001), 'the willingness to sacrifice a child with mental retardation in order to preserve the family was not in itself surprising, given prevailing assumptions about the worthlessness of these children's lives' (cited in Castles, 2004: 361). For children under six, the rate of new admissions to public institutions for mental retardation doubled between 1945 and 1955 (Castles, 2004). This was a different story to physically-disabled adults. As a result of World War Two and the Korean conflict, special veterans' legislation continued to be enacted under Eisenhower's Administration (1953–61), with primary emphasis on assisting ex-service persons to adjust from military to civilian life.

In the 1950s, parents of children with intellectual disabilities began to organise to provide opportunities for their children other than institutionalisation. The Association of Friends and Parents of the Mentally Retarded, now The Arc, was one of the first such parent organisations that began to open the doors of large institutions. Parents who founded and joined these groups were primarily young mothers and, to a lesser extent, fathers whose children were just reaching school age (Castles 2004). Early advocacy efforts focused on education for their children. Generally however their voice was lost in the broader and more vociferous 'Disability Movement' made up of mostly physically disabled young men. The eugenics movement had encouraged fears that individuals with intellectual disabilities would behave in dangerous ways, or become criminals or sexual deviants as they reached adolescence (Castles, 2004). However, the credibilty and power of the eugenics movement and of the Breeders' Association rapidly diminished as the Nazi atrocities became known (Smith, 2006). Families received a pivotal victory in 1954 in *Brown v. Board of Education,* which affirmed the right of all citizens to an equal education. Parents were able to demand that their children with disabilities be educated, preferably in the same schools as non-disabled children (Evans, 1983).

Better disability benefits came in the mid-1950s. The scope of the basic national social insurance system was significantly broadened in 1956 through the addition of *Social Security Disability Insurance (SSDI)*. Benefits were provided for severely disabled workers aged 50 or older and for adult disabled siblings of deceased or retired workers. In 1958, the *Social Security Act* was further amended to provide benefits for *dependents* of disabled workers. However, in the late 1950s, surveys of parents at 'mental retardation' clinics and in parent's groups found half of all parents had been instructed by their doctors to immediately institutionalise their child, with the proportion much higher when the child was diagnosed with Down Syndrome (Castles, 2004).

Rights and Entitlements Expansion (1960–1979)

Major expansion of welfare expenditure began to take place in the 1960s, and continued into the mature post-war Keynesian corporatist settlement of the 1960s and 1970s. Also, no other period saw the roots of so many changes including rights, mainstreaming, advocacy, individual plans, interdisciplinary teams, normalisation, and the roots of deinstitutionalisation (Smith, 2006). In 1961 President John F. Kennedy established the President's Panel on Mental Retardation, which went on to make a number of significant recommendations, many of which were incorporated into legislation. For example, for the first time states were required to produce comprehensive plans for the development of improved community services with the *Mental Retardation Facilities and Community Mental Health Centers Construction Act* of 1963 (implemented in 1965) (Simons and Watson, 1999). This provided funding for the formation of the first university-affiliated facilities and programs which were developed and funded to provide education, service, and research to individuals with mental retardation and their families. Kennedy had also planned an ambitious legislative program for the last year of his term but was assassinated on November 1963. Much of his agenda was continued however between 1964–1966 when Lyndon Johnson took office. His immediate priority was to enshrine the *Civil Rights Act* (1964) which outlawed discrimination on the basis of race in public accommodations and employment, as well as in federally assisted programs. Although disability or family caregivers were not on the agenda, it became a model for subsequent disability non-discrimination legislation.

More generally, the 1960s ushered in an era of federal support, professional development, better services, and increased public understanding to enhance the lives of persons with intellectual disabilities and their families (Nehring 2004). Lejeune et al. had by now published that an extra small chromosome was present in individuals with Down's syndrome (1959) and by 1963, geneticists had discovered other structural chromosal abnormalities as reasons for mental retardation. References to 'mongolism' therefore declined, which reduced the stigma for families. In 1965, Senator Robert Kennedy visited Willowbrook institution for the mentally retarded and publicised the scandalous conditions that existed there, calling it a 'snake pit'. Equally provoking was Burton Blatt's visit to Willowbrook with professional photographer Fred Kaplan later that year, which resulted in a famous photographic essay, *Christmas in Purgatory* (1974), on the atrocious conditions.

Under Johnson's leadership, legislation was also passed in 1965 creating the two most fundamental Acts in health care in US history; *Medicare* and *Medicaid*. The Democrats ruled both houses at this time and these acts have subsequently been referred to by some commentators as the 'flowerchild of health policy' (Oberlander, 2003). The Medicare program has since provided for the medical needs of persons aged 65 or older and some people under age 65 with disabilities. It has primarily covered acute care costs and has not been considered a major payer for long-term care (Family Caregiver Alliance, 2003b). Medicaid on the other hand was set up to meet the long-term service needs of people with disabilities and chronically ill. It has since been a federal-state funding partnership with three coverage programs in one: (1) insurance coverage for low-income children and pregnant women, (2) additional coverage for low-income elders on Medicare, and (3) acute and long-term care coverage for people with disabilities and frail elders. Under federal law, Medicaid was meant to provide coverage for rehabilitation and other services so that people could attain and retain capability for independence or self-care (Winchester and Frydman, 2003). Since its inception, Medicaid is structured and operated somewhat differently in each state and the District of Columbia. Each state decides how to operate its program within federal guidelines, establishing or influencing the reimbursement rate, amount, scope, and duration of home health and personal care benefits offered (Newcomer et al., 2001).

When first enacted, Federal Medicaid funding was available only when the person was placed in an institutional setting, with few avenues for securing Medicaid dollars to support individuals in their homes (Smith, et al., 2000: 1). This was because policymakers concentrated primarily on the sickest and most disabled members of this population, due to their extensive service needs, many of whom had major cognitive problems and limited decision-making capacity (Batavia, 2003: 2). In 1970, half of all home care was supported by private third-party payers (not including private health insurance) and primarily philanthropic organisations. From less than $1 billion in 1966, Medicaid grew to a program whose expenditures were to reach $318 billion in financial year (FY) 2008 (NASBO, 2009).

Medicaid eligibility rules fall into two basic sets: *categorical* and *financial*. The categorical set defines particular categories of persons for whom Federal law permits coverage (elderly, blind, or disabled). The financial eligibility is deeply rooted in two federally financed programs of cash assistance to help support low-income individuals and families: the *Aid to Families with Dependent Children* (AFDC) program, which provided income support for low-income families with children and *Supplemental Security Income*, introduced later (discussed below). The person must also be unable to work, or have a level of earning considered by regulation as evidence of one's inability to engage in 'substantial gainful activity'.

There is also a 'spend down option' available in most States, allowing an individual to use incurred/unpaid medical bills to 'spend down' the difference between their income and the income limit to become eligible (Kaiser Commission on Medicaid and the Uninsured, 2001: 2).

The next five years of Medicaid's history were heavily influenced by major amendments to the *Social Security Acts* (SSA) that were passed by Congress in late 1971 and 1972. The 1972 amendments created the *Supplemental Security Income* (SSI) program, which federalised existing State cash assistance programs for persons with disabilities (to which the state could add additional monies) (Klemm, 2000: 107). SSI has since been a means-tested programme for people with disabilities, requiring that the individual's income and assets fall below a minimum standard.

Prepaid health care remained a minor phenomenon until the 1970s, largely as a result of the strong resistance from the American Medical Association. In the late 1960s and early 1970s, politicians and interest groups promoted various proposals for reforming the nation's healthcare system. Issues of cost containment, coverage for the uninsured, access to services for the poor and minorities, consumer rights, efficient delivery systems, and more were all on the agenda. During the Nixon administration (1969–74), the *Health Maintenance Act* (1973) was signed into law, which established 'Health Maintenance Organizations' (HMOs), which are group practices to provide prepaid health plans to enrolled members and for their care to be arranged from a designated provider network (Tufts Managed Care Institute, 1998). However, these have remained limited in their ability to cater for the needs of people with disabilities, as these models often offer too restrictive a menu of service options, and enrolees cannot use their Medicaid dollars to pay for services outside the remit of their Managed Care provider. Similarly, managed care organisations are unlikely to have well-developed relationships with providers of the specialised ancillary services that persons with disabilities use, for example, wheelchair manufacturers and personal care attendants.

The disability movement had at this time become quite a sizeable lobby group, made up of mostly people with physical disabilities from the war efforts. Intensive campaigning against discrimination gained a shift in policy designed to reduce segregation and remove social and environmental barriers, as evidenced in the *Architectural Barriers Act* (1968). This mandated that federally constructed buildings and facilities be accessible to people with physical disabilities. This Act is generally considered to be the first-ever federal disability rights legislation. In 1972 Paralyzed Veterans of America, the National Paraplegia Foundation, and Richard Heddinger filed a law-suit to force the Washington Metropolitan Area Transit Authority to incorporate access into their design for a new, multibillion-dollar subway system in Washington, D.C. Their eventual victory became a landmark in the struggle for accessible public transit (Disability Social History Project, 2003).

This period also saw improvements in the independent living movement. With the *Rehabilitation Act* (1973), severely disabled persons who were judged not potentially employable were made eligible to receive such services as needed so as to enable them to live independently. The public sector rehabilitation programs are primarily federally funded under the guidance of the Rehabilitation Services Administration (RSA). Besides administering the funds which go to the state rehabilitation agencies, the RSA has funds for innovations in service delivery, improving relations with employers, research, demonstration programs and training (Pfeiffer, 2001). Although many persons with disabilities have benefited greatly from rehabilitation, its ethos at this time was largely focused on sheltered employment.

The de-institutionalisation movement also started in the 1970s with the growing discourse of normalisation. Throughout the decade, institutions and community services operated as parallel service systems for people with intellectual disabilities (Metzel 2004). However, the conditions of many institutions caring for those with an intellectual disability began to increasingly come under public scrutiny. In the US, in 1972 Geraldo Rivera, made a TV programme which exposed the appalling conditions of those with an intellectual disability in two large institutions in New York. Many (see Mansell and Ericsson, 1996) considered this the single most important event to give impetus to the development away from institutional services. The emphasis on normalisation began to replace the earlier eugenic ideas. However, with community care only in its infancy, the majority of institutionalised patients were simply rehoused in Intermediary Care Facilities for the Mentally Retarded (ICFs/MR) or group homes.

By mid-1970s, family caregiver support in general, and respite care in particular, had never been the focus of US welfare or health policy. However with the inception of deinstitutionalisation, caregiver support programs first started appearing in the statutes of several states. The first state respite programs, along with other caregiver support services, were created in the 1970s (Silberberg, 2001: 1) with one of the oldest programs focused on family support for the developmentally disabled population: Washington's *Family Support Program* in 1975.

The move towards greater recognition of carers continued with the establishment of Family Caregiver Alliance in 1977, as a public voice for caregivers, offering them assistance with education, services, research and advocacy. Starting as a small task force of families and community leaders in San Francisco, they came together to create support services for those struggling to provide long term care for a loved one who did not 'fit' into traditional health systems: adults with Alzheimer's disease, stroke, Parkinson's, traumatic brain injuries and other debilitating disorders. The diagnoses were different, but the families shared common challenges: isolation, lack of information, few community resources, and drastic changes in family roles. The task force's early efforts had three lasting results: the formation of Family Caregiver Alliance; the genesis of California's statewide network of Caregiver Resource Centers; and the beginnings of a national movement to recognise the immense contribution of family caregivers to the long-term health care needs of those ill, disabled, or elderly (Family Caregiver Alliance, 2003a).

These were quite in contrast to the direction the disability movement was going from the mid- to late-1970s, concentrating on empowering the disabled person rather than the carer. In 1977, a group of disabled people took over the San Francisco offices of the Health, Education, and Welfare Department to protest Secretary Joseph Califano's refusal to sign meaningful regulations for Section 504 of the *Rehabilitation Act*. Section 504 is a civil rights law which prohibits discrimination against individuals with disabilities. The action became the longest sit-in of a federal building to date lasting almost a month. The historic demonstrations were successful and the 504 regulations were finally signed (Disability Social History Project, 2003). The demonstrations helped galvanise the disability community nationwide.

Another landmark was a ruling by District Judge Raymond Broderick in 1977 that keeping people with 'mental retardation' in institutions was a violation of their constitutional rights in the landmark class action suit against the Penhurst School for the Mentally Retarded in Pennsylvania. Lawsuits were also filed on behalf of the people living in institutions and their relatives in a dozen states, including New York (Willowbrook), Michigan (Plymouth), Alabama (Partlow). These early lawsuits were designed to force states to improve the institutions by adequately funding them, hiring and training more staff, and providing services that would help people achieve their potential. The Pennhurst case however, and all subsequent lawsuits, transformed into judgments which claimed that no amount of money could remedy the obvious facts of isolation and segregation – which they claimed led directly to abuse and neglect (Conroy, 1996). Rather than improving the institutions, they ruled that segregation should be abolished and people should be served in communities and neighbourhoods just like anyone else. In the Pennhurst case, every person would have to be accorded a new home and a new life in communities around Pennsylvania. The subsequent surge of litigation also spurred the transformation of the movement for fair and humane treatment into a true civil rights movement. The inclusion of Section 504 within the *Rehabilitation Act* of 1973 provided the legislative foundation for later litigation – it was worded in the same way as the *Civil Rights Act*: 'Nondiscrimination Under Federal Grants and Programs'. It also brought the concepts of de-institutionalisation and normalisation into the vocabulary of services for people with intellectual disabilities. Unfortunately, early support from states for these concepts was sparse and implementation varied significantly from one state to the next (Evans, 1983).

These positive landmarks in family caregiving and disability were overshadowed in the late 1970s when inflation skyrocketed under President Carter. For many Americans, the economic, social and political trends of the previous two decades, which culminated in the economic downturn and inflation of the Carter years, engendered a mood of disillusionment. Republicans, long out of power at the Federal level, were well positioned to exploit this new mood. It was a time when many Americans were receptive to their message of limited government, strong national defence and the protection of traditional values (KSAH, 2002).

Retrenchment and Expansion (1980–1990)

In the 1980s, the US experienced two short sharp recessions, known as the 'double-dip' recessions of 1980–82 and 1987 (Boyd and Nathan, 2003). The first recession marked the early years of President Reagan's presidency (1981–89). Reagan's program was rooted in his belief that the nation would prosper if the power of the private economic sector was unleashed. He was also intent on promoting his neo-liberal agenda in health care, with doctrines of structural adjustment, privatisation, deregulation, and market based development. He believed state intervention in the market should be minimised on the grounds that it undermines the efficiency of markets, and that only minimal state intervention was necessary to ensure the fairness of business practice. His administration began to recognise Health Maintenance Organizations (HMOs) as cost containment entitlement programs and started to set up Medicaid and Medicare HMOs. It is also worth noting that the two programs became co-ordinated under the one roof by the Health Care Financing Administration (HCFA). Employers came to look upon managed care as a less expensive yet comprehensive and high quality form of insurance to offer their employees. By the mid-1980s, HMOs were starting to be known as profit making companies, and in 1984, HMOs went public. At this stage very few carers or their recipients were enrolled but this became more dominant as they developed.

The move toward care at home was building for many years, but a pivotal moment came in 1981, when Reagan signed the *Medicaid Home and Community-Based Services (HCBS) Waiver Program* into law.[1] Prior to this legislation, Medicaid long-term care benefits were limited to institutional facilities: hospitals, nursing facilities and ICFs/MR. According to the New York Times (Fisher, 1988), President Reagan singled out a young girl Katie Beckett from Iowa at a news conference, who, as a result of Medicaid regulations had to suffer from viral encephalitis in a hospital, at a cost of $12,000 a month, rather than be allowed to be cared for at home, where it would cost $4,000 or less. This became known as the '1915 Waiver' (after the regulation it waived), or colloquily the 'Katie Beckett Waiver'. The term 'Waiver' therefore means that certain statutes, regulations, and limits on services and eligibility are waived in order to provide HCBS in the community, as long as the cost of care was no more than the institutional cost of care. From 1993, these waivers grew from $1.6bn to $14.4bn in 1998 (primarily for those with intellectual disabilities) (Smith, et al., 2000). Because of the strict eligibility rules, the disability rights movement began urging Congress to change the Medicaid program so that each recipient would be free to choose whether to receive services in an institution or at home. In essence, the Medicaid legislation still specified placement in an institution in the first instance and only offered these 'waivers' if additional categorical requirements were met.

Since this time, states have been able to determine the size, geographic location, and the target groups eligible for the waiver programs. Because of this discretion,

1 Within the established section 1915(c) of the *Social Security Act.*

the growth in waivers and expenditures has been uneven across and within states with documented differences in service access and availability (O'Shaughnessy et al., 2002: 5). States typically operate three or four waiver programs, but some states offer more. Colorado, for example, operates ten (Schneider and Garfield, 2003). Each state may offer a distinct package of services and supports to a different group of individuals under a specific HCBS waiver program (Smith et al., 2000).

By 1985, with continuing improvements in the economy, Congress embarked on a series of Medicaid expansions that continued each year through the end of the decade. The HCBS waiver legislation provided a vehicle for states, for the first time, to offer additional services not otherwise available through their Medicaid programs to serve people in their own homes and communities (Coleman et al., 2003). However, many of the expansions introduced were subject to delayed effective dates or phase-in provisions, leading to geographical disparities, thus the full effect of this era's expansions was not felt during the period (Klemm, 2000: 109).

As a result of the dominant political discourse on spending cuts, reducing the deficit etc., disabled people and their families were tired of being in a dependency trap with the government. In 1986, from limited beginnings the disability movement in the US embarked on an even more radical course than just attempting to restructure welfare, with its emphasis on securing the *rights* of disabled people. The 'National Council on the Handicapped' issued a report entitled, *Toward Independence*, which outlined the legal status of Americans with disabilities, documenting the existence of discrimination and citing the need for federal civil rights legislation. This came about from more than 20 years of powerful lobbying by disabled people and their allies. World War Two, and subsequent wars throughout the last century had contributed to a formidable lobby group made up of mostly young, physically disabled, and vociferous people. They sought to change the framework of the social debate by challenging the notion that individuals with disabilities were another special interest group requiring a set of special services. Instead, they focused on gaining equal rights to education, public transportation, social services, access to public places and employment (Chatterjee and Mitra, 1998). This led to the most significant piece of disability legislation worldwide, which is examined in the next section.

Family caregivers also continued to become more vociferous during the 1980s. An organisation called the *National Family Caregivers Association* (NFCA) was established to educate, support and empower family caregivers and speak out publicly for meeting caregivers' needs (National Family Caregivers Association, 2001). Another voluntary association which took interest in caregiving issues was *The Rosalynn Carter Institute for Human Development* (RCI), formed by the former First Lady Rosalynn Carter in 1987. Through research, education, and training, the RCI began to promote the mental health and well-being of caregivers; encourage effective caregiving practices; build public awareness of caregiving needs; and advance public and social policies that enhance caring communities. Many faith-based organisations at state level also began to offer support and assistance to older persons, adults with disabilities, and family caregivers, such as the *Beatitudes Center for Developing Older Adult Resources* – an interfaith ministry in Arizona. As a result of the diversity in ethnicity and faith in the US, many caregivers look toward their own ethnic and faith groups for such support

By now there was a long, robust history of state-operated 'family support' programs. The aim of these was to provide supports that benefited *both* the individual and the family and, thereby, contribute to maintaining and sustaining the family unit (Smith et al., 2000: 139). While the most common source of state support was general funds, other sources included casino tax revenues and tobacco settlement funds (Silberberg, 2001). A range of state agencies administered caregiver support programs, including Departments of Aging, health services, and developmental disabilities services. State Departments of Aging, the most common administrative agency (19 programs in 13 states), developed programs such as caregiver education, training and respite that meet the caregiving and long-term needs of the care recipient (Fox-Grage et al., 2001).

State approaches varied greatly however, the reality being that few states had a consistent package of caregiver supports. Instead, they had a range of programs with different eligibility requirements, divergent funding sources and varied funding levels. The use of separate agencies to handle different aspects of care management – such as determining coverage eligibility, authorising payments, and advocating for clients – led to geographic disparity which made it difficult for persons with disabilities and their families to negotiate a complex service maze (Kaiser Commission on Medicaid and the Uninsured, 2001).

The Rise of Disability Rights (1990–1992)

In July, 1990, President George Bush signed in the *Americans with Disabilities Act* (ADA) into law. This was a landmark federal legislation guaranteeing people with disabilities the same rights to employment and access to public facilities as other citizens. A key point in its implementation however was that the costs were transferred to business. Many have argued that the reason the Act became law was more to do with the economic rationality underpinning it than any moral concerns (Drake, 1999). The ADA presented an opportunity to turn the corner on policies promoting welfare-like dependence and to develop supports for independence in the context of working, living and recreating in the mainstream. In this sense implementing the ADA was seen as an opportunity to contribute to an improved economy. When persons with disabilities give up public subsidies for jobs, they become taxpayers; thus contributing directly to public treasuries.

It has been recognised as the most comprehensive disability legislation in the world. Building on earlier protections under Section 504 of the *Rehabilitation Act* of 1973, the ADA extended anti-discrimination protections well beyond prior law, reaching private employment, publicly funded services and public accommodations, including services operated by private entities (Rosenbaum, 2001). Prior to the ADA, disability rights policies had been criticised for being based almost exclusively on federal spending levels. This was identified as causing confusion and inequity in the implementation of disability rights polices by state and local governments (Percy, 2001: 248). Geographically then, it was determined that not all states could be counted on to enact comprehensive non-discrimination statutes. Therefore, the legislation moved disability policy towards a national, centralised position. The ADA language went to unusual lengths to specify coverage of state and local governments. Despite Republicans being against the creation of new federal mandates, it gained unusual support in Congress and in the White House.

Using a broad definition of disability, the Act accorded extensive rights to disabled people under four main sections (see Drake, 1999: 105). The first part outlawed discrimination against disabled people in public and private sector employment. Disabled people who could perform the 'essential functions' of a job were protected by the legislation. Companies were prohibited from discriminating against such candidates and had to set in train 'readily achievable', 'reasonable' accommodations to the workplace to facilitate disabled employees (Blakemore and Drake, 1996). The second part focused on access to public services and transport: public bodies were compelled to make 'reasonable' changes to rules, policies and practices, and had to remove physical barriers, or provide auxiliary aids, in order to ensure that their services were usable by disabled people. This meant all new public service vehicles had to be accessible (Blakemore and Drake, 1996). The third part required access for disabled people to educational, recreational and leisure facilities such as schools, cinemas and shops. Education was a particularly important area. Le Plante et al. (1997) argue that employment chances have been blighted by low skills among disabled Americans, and a key reason for this has been lack of vocational training and restricted access to mainstream schools and colleges.

The final part detailed the enforcement structures of the Act and the avenues of redress available to disabled people where employers or service providers failed to comply with the law. The Act has been enforced by an Equal Employment Opportunities Commision and by designated state agencies. One of the main strands of argument against the introduction of similar legislation in Britain or Ireland has been concern about the cost of implementation. Higgens (1992) recorded similar anxieties in America leading to substantial resistance by businesses and corporations. In the event however, the implementation of the ADA has led neither to excessive expenditure or litigation nor to commercial bankruptcies (Drake, 1999: 107).

While the ADA effectively targeted those who could achieve independence with these mandates, it made less provision for those still needing extensive support to live semi-independently. Title II of the Act ruled that State and local governments 'must provide programs and services in an integrated setting, unless separate or different measures are necessary to ensure equal opportunity'. However, because of its strong focus on access for people who were 'work ready', many have felt that those who needed long-term care including the elderly, and people with mental illness, or intellectual disabilities were left behind due to the strong non-discrimination focus of the ADA and not heard in the disability rights movement. Furthermore, this has had huge implications on families, as the majority of the care support work has fallen on informal care to facilitate this independent model of living. In terms of outcomes of these public policies, the literature on assistance versus insurance contains some findings that people with intellectual disabilities and those who are profoundly disabled make up the largest beneficiaries of assistance more than others. The explosive growth of SSI shows that despite the legislation, the demand for long-term care will continue to exist (Chatterjee and Mitra, 1998).

The Clinton Aspirations (1993–2000)

In the early 1990s, George Bush was unable to withstand discontent from the faltering economy and strained state budgets. He was succeeded in 1993 by William J. Clinton. The new Administration started by increasing income and sales taxes to ameliorate the 1990–91 downturn. Clinton decided early in his term of office that debt reduction, rather than tax cuts, was the best way to preserve economic growth. By cutting federal spending, creating millions of new jobs, and reducing the deficit, he wanted to restore economic opportunity and security (Riley, 2002).

He entered office with a wide-ranging agenda, appointing his wife to head a task force to deal with health-care reform to try to make health care available for all. The *Health Security Act* (1993) included universal health care coverage, prescription drug benefits for the elderly, increased public health initiatives, and purchasing alliances to expand employer-sponsored benefits (Levin-Epstein, 2000). As a whole, the plan unceremoniously failed however, as the administration failed to achieve universal coverage. Most observers say it was the massive cost of the Clinton proposal – or at least its perceived cost – that, more than anything else, made it fail (Levin-Epstein, 2000). Further, the American Medical Association was still resistant against State involvement in health care.

However, the spirit of the administration's effort to overhaul health care delivery lived on and, in some cases, pieces of the 1993–94 proposal took on new life in the form of state law (Levin-Epstein, 2000: 3). A period of economic growth from 1992 encouraged this process, as the nature of the growth was especially good for state finances. This came about from their response to the weakened economy and the 1990–91 downturn, by increasing taxes substantially, leading to a nominal state revenue growth rate of 90 per cent between 1990 and 2000, (Boyd and Nathan, 2003: 13–14).

During his Presidency, the number of caregivers, according to the Survey of Income and Program Participation (1996), conducted by the Census Bureau, was estimated to be 24.1 million (Arno et al., 1999). In terms of long-term care, the administration proposed a $6 billion five-year package to begin to address the long-term care needs of persons with disabilities and their families. By explicitly recognising that family members were the core long-term care providers in the US care system, this initiative opened a long-overdue policy discussion (Arno et al., 1999). Using a very high federal participation rate, Clinton encouraged states to establish more HCBS programs for disabled people of all ages. The entitlement was to an assessment and a care plan; the states were free to spend their money and the federal government matched this up to a capped amount to provide the care needed (Friedland, 1997: 149).

President Clinton also established a \$1000 tax credit for people in need of long term home or institutional care (Cantwell, 2001). Although it may have eased the burden of certain existing long term care costs, it failed however to provide enhanced incentives to purchase long-term care insurance. Furthermore, only a small percentage actually qualified for such a tax credit. The financial incentive was regarded as insufficient to cause large numbers of people to buy such insurance (Friedland, 1997). He also established a \$125m annual grant to the states to fund programs that would provide information, counselling, and training to home caregivers. Interestingly, he made \$10m available to instruct Medicare beneficiaries about the *limitations* of long-term care coverage under Medicare; surveys had found that as many as 60 per cent of the elderly and disabled were unaware that Medicare did not cover most long term care costs (Cantwell, 2001: 268).

The most prominent workplace initiative aimed at supporting family caregivers came about around this time also; the *Family and Medical Leave Act* (1993). It required employers with more than 50 workers to permit employees to take up to 12 weeks of unpaid leave to care for a family member. These tight restrictions however have made the scheme very difficult for family members to receive, and mirrors similar workplace benefits in Ireland. Some employers and unions have gone further by establishing 'family-friendly' programs to reduce conflict between work and family caregiving, including flexible scheduling; part-time work options with benefits; information and referral services; and caregiver support groups. Financial benefits like dependent care assistance programs and reimbursement accounts are less often available (Stone, 1999).

While these developments were taking place, Medicaid long-term care spending continued to grow throughout the 1990s, straining state budgets (O'Shaughnessy et al., 2002: 1). In response to this, in 1996, Congress passed legislation which had a major negative impact on eligibility for Medicaid and for family caregivers. The *Personal Responsibility and Work Opportunity Reconciliation Act* was a federal 'reform' law which brought new emphasis to work among parents receiving welfare and discouraged families from relying on public assistance. It changed 'Aid to Families with Dependent Children' (AFDC) to a new program called 'Temporary Assistance for Needy Families' (TANF). Formerly, under AFDC the disabled person and the carer were automatically eligible for Medicaid, but now individuals had to qualify for the program separately (Skinner et al., 2002) Although adults with disabilities typically qualify for Medicaid based on their eligibility for Supplemental Security Income (SSI), their carers were now made to apply separately, and many failed to qualify because parent eligibility levels were below poverty in most states (Skinner et al., 2002). For families with disabled members these requirements led to much added financial worry. The Act effectively de-coupled Medicaid from cash assistance for low-income families (Klemm, 2000). Although requirements varied by state and family circumstance, these 'reforms' limited the time that a family could receive cash payments and required that carers enter the workforce or become more 'work ready' (Skinner et al., 2002: 2).

In response to fiscal crisis and to overcome the rising complexity of programs, states began to invest much time and resources into care coordination and case management in the form of 'Medicaid Managed Care'. The move toward greater Medicaid Managed Care enrolment came with the *Balanced Budget Act (BBA)* (1997). Most states converted major portions of their Medicaid programs from fee-for-service to managed care models. Proponents of Medicaid reform through managed care argued that it would control cost growth and create a 'medical home', offering Medicaid beneficiaries better and more consistent access to primary care and coordination of services (Haslanger, 2003). However this has been increasingly challenged given the cost growth in the US health care system In any case, the government gave states the option of setting up Medicaid managed care programs without the waivers that were usually required for such programs, opening up the market for private companies such as the *Medical Case Management of America, Inc*. (MCMA) to provide case management services. Of the total Medicaid enrolment in the United States in 2004, approximately 60 per cent were receiving Medicaid benefits through managed care.

As discussed earlier, managed care however, has typically not been part of the Medicaid program's disability-oriented service array. Indeed, some disability advocacy groups have spoken out publicly against enrolment in MCOs (see Tanenbaum and Hurley, 1995). According to their paper, where it has been initiated, the results have been tentative and mixed. Early demonstration programs in Santa Barbara, California, and in Minneapolis came into conflict with both advocacy groups and managed care plans, specifically regarding providers' readiness to serve disabled populations. Despite this, Medicaid managed care for persons with disabilities is still under active consideration in many states. The care coordination inherent in managed care was conceived as a means of assisting families in navigating through complex Medicaid managed care systems in obtaining information and access to services (Wunderlich and Kohler, 2001). Because beneficiaries with disabilities typically require the services of multiple physicians and other providers, some MCOs are mobilising their referral network through partnerships with the consumer, the consumer's family, advocacy groups, Centers for Independent Living and other state agencies (Smith et al., 2000: 108). In theory, this has meant that care management can develop networks for ongoing support, monitor the care recipients' situation on an ongoing basis, and adjust the service package as needed (Smith et al., 2000). By 2004, Medicaid Managed Care was available for adults with disabilities in 66 per cent of US counties, up from 43 per cent in 1996 (Burns, 2009).

However the reality for most citizens was that in 1997, more Americans were uninsured than at any other time in the previous two decades, yet the unemployment rate in 1999 was the nation's lowest since 1969 (Case et al., 2002). Explanations from health policy research focused on rising costs of coverage, growing service-sector and part-time employment, declining unionisation, segregation of high- and low-wage workers into different firms and error in the measurement of coverage (Case et al., 2002). This has meant that families largely were paying out of pocket and in many cases had to continue to pay until they reached income levels low enough for Medicaid eligibility. At the same time, states varied significantly in their rates of using Medicaid dollars on the provision of Home- and Community-Based waiver services. In 1997, for example, that share was less than 8 per cent in half the states. In the same year, however, five states spent more than 20 per cent of their Medicaid long-term care resources on home and community services, with Oregon and New York at 40 to 50 per cent (Smith et al., 2000: 8–9).

In January 1999, the Health Care Financing Administration (HCFA) thoroughly revised and updated the Agency's guidelines concerning coverage of personal care services. The use of Activities of Daily Living (ADL) measures as the basis for determining how carers become eligible for both private and publicly funded benefits had become a contentious issue (Reinhard, 2001). Although eligibility criteria for state supported services for family caregivers varied substantially across the states, the propensity to frame needs in 'the most rudimentary acts of survival' – bathing, dressing, eating, toileting – represented in the care recipient's ADLs was a problem for caregivers who did more than help with baths and feeding (Reinhard, 2001). It was estimated that as much as 80 per cent of the caregiving responsibilities remained unexplained in this framework (Reinhard, 2001). The new Agency's guidelines made it clear that personal care services may span provision of assistance not only with ADLs but also with Instrumental Activities of Daily Living (IADLs) – such as personal hygiene, light housework, laundry, meal preparation, transportation, grocery shopping, using the telephone, medication management, and money management. However neither the statutory provisions nor the revised Federal regulations and State Medicaid guidelines dictated that a state *must* change the scope of its pre-1993 personal care coverage (Boyd and Nathan, 2003: 27).

Despite all the talk about public HCBS, nursing home expenditures still accounted for the vast majority of Medicaid spending. By the year 2000, it still appeared that private health insurance was largely not available, affordable or adequate for families with intellectually disabled members. This has been due to its expense and the limitations on coverage. In a Kaiser Commissioned study, families with private insurance often were required to make steep co-payments and were not necessarily better off unless they also had Medicaid coverage (Skinner et al., 2002: 3). According to Stone (2001: 102), the individual policy market for disability-type policies had little growth from 1991 to 2001, probably because of the higher premiums associated with this product relative to indemnity plans.

Towards the end of the Clinton Administration, community care for adults with intellectual disabilities went through another major transformation. A case was brought to the U.S. Supreme Court in 1999[2] by two women who had been institutionalised, despite the fact that professionals had determined that they could be appropriately treated in a community setting. The *Olmstead* case as it became known was a landmark in disability legislation. The Supreme Court held that the medically unjustifiable institutionalisation of persons with disabilities constituted a form of discrimination and therefore a violation of the *Americans with Disabilities Act* (1990). It ruled that when a state's own medical professionals reasonably conclude that an individual is able to reside in the community, the state must make *reasonable modifications* to furnish community services in the most integrated setting unless the state can prove that to do so would require a *fundamental alteration* of its program (Rosenbaum, 2001). In essence, *Olmstead* required that states plan for and undertake two basic reforms: the broad and complex task of restructuring existing programs and services in order to promote community integration, and the establishment of an individualised assessment process to design community placements (Rosenbaum, 2001).

In terms of state efforts, the ruling has stimulated many States to increase community-based alternatives to institutionalisation for people with disabilities of all ages, particularly people with intellectual disabilities. Evidence from state websites suggest that most states are moving ahead with planning and that in general states' planning efforts are broad based in their involvement of community stakeholders, public agencies and programs. Following the decision, a state could decide to make increased use of the Medicaid program to increase both the amount and share of its resources going to HCBS (Smith, et al., 2000: 8). Whether the subsequent planning processes reflected the full range of issues raised by the decision has been unclear (Rosenbaum, 2001). In any case, sweeping decisions such as this one often take years to 'filter through' the health and social service systems because of difficulties interpreting the full meaning of the decision and the complexities of modifying the ongoing operations of public programs to achieve consistency with the goal of maximum integration (Rosenbaum, 2001).

The implications of the Supreme Court's *Olmstead* decision for family caregivers remain unclear. The emphasis of services for people with intellectual disabilities is now copper-fastened on reintegrating them back into the community. Of particular concern to family caregivers may be the ability of programs to pay families to provide support and assistance normally furnished by agencies and personal assistants (Fox-Grage et al., 2001). As states continue to develop their state plans, family caregivers of people with intellectual disabilities need to be integrally involved.

---

2 *Olmstead vs. L.C.*, Ruling made in June 22, 1999, Georgia.

Increasing Recognition of Carers (2001–2002)

George W. Bush was sworn into office January 20, 2001, after a campaign in which he outlined sweeping proposals to modernise Social Security and Medicare, provide tax relief, and encourage faith-based and community organisations to work with government. Since Clinton and the *Olmstead* ruling, both federal and state governments began directing greater attention to the problems of family caregivers. Under Bush, major federal legislative, judicial and administrative actions have begun to change the landscape for family caregivers and affected state policy directly and indirectly. At the Federal level, several recent laws and rulings have promised to increase funding for support services for family caregivers and for stimulating state innovations in long-term care.

At the Federal level, on June 18, 2001, President Bush issued *Executive Order 13217* as a response to *Olmstead* affirming the US's commitment to community-based alternatives and programs that foster independence and participation in the community (Rosenbaum, 2001). In addition, to support informal caregivers, the Administration implemented the *National Family Caregiver Support Program* (NFCSP) under the *Older Americans Act* (OAA) Amendments of 2000. It received broad, bipartisan support and stands as the most significant legislative accomplishment to date on behalf of family caregivers in the US (Stone, 1999). It was modelled in large part after successful programs in States such as California, New Jersey, Wisconsin and Pennsylvania (Takamura, 2001, cited in Silberberg, 2001). Through a national network of state and Area Agencies on Aging (AAAs), the program provides information to caregivers about available counselling, support groups, training, and other services. In addition, the program provides respite care to temporarily relieve caregivers. Swift approval of its first year funding at the full authorisation level ($125m) demonstrated that family caregiving was now a legitimate political constituency issue in Washington (Whitehouse, 2001). In FY 2002 funding was increased to $141.5m and the proposed level in FY 2003 was $160.5. In releasing the money in formula grants to the states, the Administration on Aging provided the most minimal of guidelines, allowing the states to move forward quickly to expand existing caregiver programs operating under the *Older Americans Act*.

Although an extremely modest proposal, it was the first time that some states explicitly served family caregivers as an identified 'client'. A key development since the passage of the NFSCP has been the paradigm shift in long-term care, with family care being put on the national agenda (Stone, 1999: 10). The NFCSP provides, for the first time, some minimal support to moderate-income families who are not Medicaid eligible and for whom there are limited or no state-funded caregiver support programs. Middle income families – who are above the eligibility limit for most other publicly funded programs – often cannot afford to pay for needed respite and other caregiver supports. Consequently, middle-income caregivers are often the most at risk for impoverishment (Fox-Grage et al., 2001).

Supporting caregivers directly for their services still remains a contentious issue however. On one hand, several states fund significant multifaceted caregiver support programs from their state general revenues (California, Pennsylvania, Washington) (Fox-Grage et al., 2001). The Caregiver Resource Centers in California are regarded as being a good practice model.[3] Various Medicaid 'Family and Caregiver Support' options are also available across states. Many offer training and education services to caregivers, to strengthen their ability to meet the needs of the person they are caring for (Smith et al., 2000). States also offer respite services under Medicaid waivers to provide relief to the caregiver. However, respite services cannot be furnished if they principally benefit the 'family unit'. While they may indirectly benefit the family, they are provided directly to the beneficiary (Smith et al., 2000). On the other hand, carer support varies significantly, with the *Survey of Fifteen States' Caregiver Support Programs: Final Report* (Feinberg and Pilisuk, 1999) finding that the number of program sites in the 15 states varied dramatically from six to 600, reflecting differences in state size, configuration of program, budget, and interpretation of the term 'site' (e.g., regional/county offices, or local-level provider contracts). This is likely to continue as the ability of states to pilot new programs increased in August 2001, when the Secretary issued a new set of guidelines for section 1115 waivers to give states additional flexibility with respect to Medicaid benefits design. Section 1115 waivers are granted for 'experimental, pilot or demonstration projects' (Mann, 2002).

Paying caregivers directly for their services still remains a problematic issue. Federal Medicaid law allows family members to become paid caregivers unless they are legally responsible for the care of an individual (i.e., spouses and parents/guardians of children). However, states have the option to pay even these family members under certain exceptional circumstances. For example, they may be paid for providing skilled nursing services (for which there is no presumption that the service would 'normally' be provided free). There is no Federal requirement that family members provide some minimum amount of care as a condition of service eligibility. Nor is there any stipulation that services may not be furnished if a family caregiver is present. However, states can and do take into account the *amount* of informal care available to an individual. If a person needs 40 hours of support per week and family members are available, able, and willing to provide 20 hours, for example, then only 20 hours of paid supports will be authorised. In practical terms, assessment of the need for paid supports may focus on specific tasks that an family caregiver is unable to perform (Smith et al., 2000).

There is also much debate at state level over whether caregiver support programs should stand on their own or be part of larger long term care programs (Silberberg, 2001). In a FCA study (1999), most states favoured the latter approach. Even those who favoured the former approach, however, saw a need for coordination between caregiver support and long-term care initiatives (Feinberg and Pilisuk, 1999). In a later FCA study (2002), both state officials and stakeholders were asked whether

3 See CACRs website: http://www.cacrc.org.

family and informal caregivers were 'recognised' as a central component of a comprehensive long-term care system. In all but one state (Pennsylvania), key informants within the state disagreed substantially on this question. State officials generally believed that family caregivers were recognised, whereas most key stakeholders did not believe this was the case. Stakeholders typically held the view that family caregivers were neither adequately recognised nor supported in their state's long-term care system. Viewing family caregivers as a 'consumer' or 'client' population is therefore a relatively new concept for many states. As a result of the NFCSP, family caregivers were typically viewed as a 'new constituency'. Some states (Hawaii, Maine, Texas) found this paradigm shift challenging. They identified the tension between serving the care recipient, who is the traditional client in the long-term care system, and addressing the family caregivers' needs as distinct but related to the needs of the care recipient (Fox-Grage et al., 2001). Programs serving a population with intellectual disabilities were more likely to indicate that either the *family caregiver* is the client or that *both* the person with disabilities and the caregiver are clients and eligible for program services. Programs for people with physical disabilities were more likely to be 'consumer directed' (Feinberg and Pilisuk, 1999: 18). This follows similar logic to that of the ADA, where the person with a physical disability is assumed to have the capacity to make their own choices.

Overall then, care management still is primarily focused on the care recipient, and generally fails to address the caregiver's needs. According to Fox-Grage et al. (2001), states fail to promote a 'family systems' philosophy and should design long-term care that includes both the care recipient and the family caregiver as legitimate 'clients'. In their study, only 23 per cent of state officials identified the family caregiver as their primary client, and the programs they administered were typically state funded with explicit mandates to serve family and informal caregivers. Generally though, most assessment instruments to determine the care plan for the person with disabilities do not uniformly assess the needs and situation of the family caregiver.

In view of this failure to assess caregivers needs, in a national cross-section survey on caregivers (Maryam et al., 2002), it was found that vulnerable caregivers were no more likely than non-vulnerable caregivers to have received help from paid support services for their care recipients, even though they were more likely to be providing higher-intensity care, and to be aged 65 years or older. Similarly, in a Kaiser study (2002) about one in five (18 per cent) said that there was a time in the past year when they needed help caring for the person but could not get it. Out of this, almost a third said that financial concerns, including the fact that insurance was not available or did not cover the particular service, was the reason they were not able to get the help they could have used. Just as many (31 per cent) reported what could be considered deficiencies in the home care system: 15 per cent said the services were not available in their area; another 9 per cent did not know who to ask for help; and 7 per cent said that they had actually been refused help by doctors or hospitals. Only 9 per cent said they had help from home care aides or nursing assistants and 17 per cent had help from visiting nurses. Caregivers also raised serious concerns about lack of information about services.

Self-Determination and Current Challenges (2002–Present)

More recently, there has been an emerging model in US discourses of care around the concept of 'self-determination' which allows people with disabilities use an individual budget to self-direct their own publicly funded, community supports and services. It gained traction as a result of earlier demonstrations[4] in the late 1990s, as well as Olmstead's preference for home and community based care options. It culminated in the *Independence Plus* initiative, unveiled in May, 2002, by the Secretary of Health and Human Services. This offered states simplified model waiver and demonstration application templates that would promote person-centered planning and self-directed service options. Importantly, this marked the Centre for Medicare and Medicaid Services (CMS's) acceptance that the self-determination pilot programs afforded people with disabilities or their families the option to direct the design and delivery of services and supports, avoid unnecessary institutionalisation, provide higher levels of satisfaction, and maximise the efficient use of community services and supports.

Interestingly, self-determination started out as a guiding principle, but the term has since been used to denote its associated programs. Many states now have developed 'self-determination programs', through a creative use of Medicaid funding, allowing people with disabilities to 'self-direct' their own supports. This means increased autonomy for persons with disabilities, increased status within the community, and at the policy and organisational level, a fairer, more equitable distribution of public funds. With this model, individuals control planning for their own support needs, with the assistance of family and friends they designate (often referred to as a circle of support). They control a sum of public money that they have the authority to spend on residential, vocational and personal needs. Independent evaluators (Conroy et al., 2002) reported an improved quality of life for the participants, and cost savings of 12 to 15 per cent, even for the most severely disabled participants. It varies significantly across the US with Wisconsin regarded as having a good practice model on the one hand, and states like Texas not offering it as an option on the other. While many families are preferring to use this method because of the freedoms involved in designing their own supports, many other families are reluctant because they feel it represents a less secure option. To

4 The two main demonstration projects have been the *Robert Wood Johnson Foundation Self-Determination* demonstrations and the *Cash and Counseling Demonstration and Evaluation* (CCDE). The latter was set up in 1998 to test the use of the cash benefit in Arkansas, New Jersey, New York and Florida. It has largely been based on the Consumer-Directed Care (CDC) model in California.

aid families in the process, many now use fiscal intermediaries to help with the paperwork involved in hiring their own attendant care workers.

Unfortunately, while this model has been gaining in popularity, the improving economy masked the seriousness of the state fiscal conditions as state revenues fell in real terms for five straight quarters up to mid-2002 (Smith et al., 2003; Boyd and Nathan, 2003). Almost like clockwork, states have been hit with budget crises cyclically at the start of every new decade. Stemming from the late 1990s fiscal crisis, nearly every state faced budget gaps beginning in FY 2002, and these gaps grew in FY 2003 (Boyd and Nathan, 2003). In the budget environment since the beginning of the FY 2003, a total of 49 states have either made plans or already acted to reduce their Medicaid spending growth (Smith et al., 2003). Nearly half of the states were turning to reducing benefits or limiting eligibility. It also looks unlikely that the money saved on nursing homes will be redirected into HCBS for adults with intellectual disabilities (Smith et al., 2003: 12). Moreover, putting constraints on Medicaid has grave consequences and effectively little, if any, cost savings because of the loss in federal matching funds; thus controlling costs through Medicaid – just one component of the health care system – is not advised (Winchester and Frydman, 2003).

As a result of these pressures, Bush's Administration made proposals in January, 2003 to restructure Medicaid. The key elements of the alternative structure include up-front fiscal relief for states and increased state flexibility over use of funds on the one hand, and capped federal funding, which replaces the open-ended entitlement to Medicaid matching funds on the other (Kaiser Commission on Medicaid and the Uninsured, 2003: 4). In states that have chosen to pursue it, the block grant ended Medicaid as an entitlement program for many beneficiaries and eliminated open-ended federal financing. In exchange, states received far more flexibility over how they could use federal funds, making the new structure essentially a block grant to be used at the states' discretion. Although states have received a welcome boost with the up-front temporary fiscal relief, the prospects for sustained fiscal assistance from the federal government are less good, in part because the federal government faces fiscal problems of its own (Boyd and Nathan, 2003).

However the Administration appears to have sustained their interest in assisting family caregivers. In 2003, the *Family Respite Care Act* passed the Senate without opposition. The Act has authorised funds for the development of lifespan respite programs at the state and local levels, the development of planned or emergency respite care services, training and recruitment of respite care workers and volunteers, and caregiver training to help make informed decisions about respite care services (Brain Injury Resource Foundation, 2003).

Throughout the latter half of the decade, the US has been facing a major demographic and labour market challenge. This has been described by Nerney (no date) as 'The Perfect Storm'. The demographics of the population means that numbers of people in request for supports will continue to increase. During fiscal year 2000, over 700,000 individuals with developmental disabilities lived at home with a family caregiver over the age of 60. A further 928,000 lived at home with a family caregiver between 41 and 59 years, meaning an even larger cohort coming behind the 700,000 (Nerney, no date). Together with a quickly shrinking workforce it is clear that the challenges facing family support mean a new and larger commitment is required.

In January 2009, George W. Bush was replaced by Barack Obama as the new president of the US. Given the growing emphasis on individualised supports, the trend towards self-determination is likely to continue under his presidency. However, it is not a magic bullet and given the challenges facing this sector, the present system requires careful and thoughtful re-design.

Conclusion

The US has followed a very particular model in terms of its landscape of disability and care support. As a result of the disability movement successfully creating a social discourse based on independence and empowerment as opposed to charity, it is an example of a rights-based model with federal and state non-discrimination legislation supporting the rights of people with disabilities in education and the workforce. Although the US health care system suffers from fragmentation and high rates of uninsured – leading many commentators to argue it is inequitable – the role of civil rights, in particular the ADA, has been important in guaranteeing equality of participation to services for those with disabilities. However, according to Drewett (1999: 120), non-discrimination legislation must be recognised as a means, not an end. While people with disabilities are (at least in theory) armed with an arsenal of legal powers, the ability of non-discrimination legislation to support people to have an active life in the community remains limited. To reflect this, this chapter focused on how family caregivers' fare within such a model.

Unfortunately, the social discourse regarding care as solely a family responsibility has largely remained. Although there is a growing movement towards 'consumer direction', empowering the family caregiver still remains in its infancy. Little consensus exists among the states about the recognition of families as a central component of a comprehensive long-term care system. Providing explicit support for family caregivers still represents somewhat of a paradigm shift (Fox-Grage et al., 2001). In general, policy makers disagree about whether or not family caregivers should be considered clients in the long-term care system and have access to their own support services.

For many years, the main direction of long-term care state policy was to support the institutionalisation of people with intellectual disabilities. As individuals with disabilities and their families began to advocate and push for greater choice and for increased opportunities to remain in their homes and communities, states begun to broaden their focus on home and community-based care services with the newly created NFCSP, Medicaid waivers, state general funds and other state funding streams. However, with personal autonomy still being characterised as a core value of American culture, the majority of support is still directly for the person with the disability (Polivka, 2001).

Most of the public policy studies examine only the impact of community care on public expenditures, ignoring costs incurred by family caregivers (Fast et al., 1998). The economic success of the shift to community care clearly depends on the transfer of responsibility from paid health care workers to unpaid family members, and on the assumption that informal care is free. As seen, the whole paradigm towards the payment of carers is very different to England, with the choice of scheme granted towards the person with the disability; once again the result of a dominant disability lobby group. While respite is available through the Medicaid HCBS Waiver Program, in principle it is not a caregiver support program; again the care recipient must be the primary beneficiary. Attempts have been made to address this with empirical evidence by the likes of Arno and Levine (1999) and Fast et al. (1998) demonstrating the costs for informal carers. It is important to remember that while the health care given to the care recipient is critically important and usually a primary concern among most healthcare providers, the health of the caregiver cannot be overlooked or minimised. Community-based nurses need to capture the opportunity to creatively and holistically plan care for caregivers (Cuellar and Butts, 1999).

Problematically, many carers or their recipients do not currently receive the support that they need. At the core of this problem is an insufficient and fragile long term care (LTC) financing structure coupled with an already weak LTC community infrastructure which will become weaker without financing (Winchester and Frydman, 2003). Medicaid is at the heart of this problem. Today it is a far different program from that in 1965. As originally conceived, it was to have functioned much like private health insurance, with service coverage focused on acute care needs, serving primarily the very poor and near poor. Over time, federal and state actions have expanded Medicaid's authority, the scope of its coverage of long-term care services, and its eligibility options for beneficiaries. By the end of its third decade, it had become the major public funder of home and community long-term care services as well as institutional long-term care (Smith et al., 2000).

As a result of incremental policymaking, combined with vast variations in how states cover long-term care, the various facets of Medicaid's financial eligibility provisions may appear to be disjointed. It is fragmented across local programs making it difficult for Medicaid officials to put together a prudent and effective package of needed care. The lack of public funding for HCBS has left such care to the private market and to voluntary philanthropic efforts. As a consequence, the availability of services varies tremendously by community (Friedland, 1997: 143). Often the caregiver is involved in battles with bureaucracy, having difficulty counting on their insurance booklets to explain the benefits covered. With the onset of managed care and the introduction of insurance case managers who authorise or deny coverage based on their interpretation of policy language, clarity about coverage is hard to obtain (Levine and Zuckerman, 2000: 134). According to Smith et al. (2000), health care professionals must strengthen their advocacy efforts with families in creating a plan of care. In particular, there are many provisions with major eligibility discontinuities – wherein a slight change in individuals' personal circumstances can result in huge differences in the kinds (and levels) of benefits they are eligible for.

The results so far from self-determination programs have shown that they can successfully serve populations with various impairments and in various age groups. (Phillips et al., 2003). However, the barriers to broad-based reform are formidable. It appears to be a sign of the times that even the strongest advocates for helping caregivers talk little about ambitious programs like federal reform. According to Levine (1998), 'small initiatives could overcome many of the problems', such as better training for caregivers, more flexibility from employers, and a greater recognition from doctors and hospitals that families are a central part of the recipients care (cited in Fisher, 1998). In general proposals for change are being formulated in response to specific problems rather than to a broad national agenda. Therefore it is characterised as having a considerable degree of decentralisation. The current guiding principle is less one of consistent individualism than what Klass has called 'decentralised social altruism' (1985). The attempt to support flexibility at the local level appears to have promoted a variability of service options that paradoxically limits, rather than enhances, choices for family caregivers (Feinberg et al., 2002). America has been described as an 'unfinished welfare state' as early as 1972 (Keigher and Stone, 1994a). Others such as Marmor et al. (1991) have called it an 'opportunity-insurance state', emphasising personal rights and freedoms over entitlements or economic assurances. This is perhaps more accurate in terms of disability care, as the patriarchal power structures at work in the US have largely taken for granted this unpaid work, and instead followed a very particular line in ensuring the personal rights and freedoms of disabled people over coherent caregiver policies.

Chapter 6
Carer's Policy in Ireland

Evidence from looking at England and the US has made it clear that the construction of social 'norms' regarding the role of family and disability has led to very distinct local practices. It was possible to trace how each nation viewed the role of the family in providing care, and the state's own responsibility in providing assistance. The structure of the welfare system and the range of rights were much more than the organisation of services or benefits; it marked how each nation viewed social and familial responsibilities as well as the social construction of disability. Although there was a common objective in both countries to maintain the care recipient's dignity and independence in their own homes for as long as possible, the discourses regarding the responsibility of 'family' differed greatly. As a result, carers were directly and indirectly affected by a significant range of different acts of legislation and restructuring policy as well as budgetary targets. The resulting material and institutional effects were premised on the discourses, ideologies, and interactions within the state at particular times.

In England, the portrayal of the family carer in mainstream society as a major national concern has constructed an altogether different material support system to that of the US. While their policies have altered with the changing economic, social, and political context of the times, the belief in the ability of the welfare state to ameliorate the problems for people with intellectual disabilities has constructed a landscape of care which has normalised the role of the family in sustaining their independence much more clearly. With this has come an equally elaborate community support system to the US, however, one which has more noticeably targeted the carer.

In the US, the dilemma of rearing a disabled person in a society grounded in values of independence and competition has haunted US family caregivers over the course of two centuries (Brockley, 2004). However, with the rise of civil rights and the disability movement after World War Two, disability became a category under which the State had to afford rights. Indirectly family caregivers were given support under the Americans with Disabilities Act (ADA) in 1990. While the discourses and policy at Federal level maintain the ideals of capitalism and independence, at the State level much of the policies are interconnected with local notions of need. At this level, progress in caregiver policy is clearly a contested term, as some states feel the family caregiver should be supported more directly than others. More generally, the landscape of care in the US has typically constructed the care recipient as the target of social support.

While carers in England get more recognition in political discourse, it is more difficult to qualitatively judge across England and the US which is the better system for carers. The US rights movement has arguably focused on the more vocal, young physically disabled population, while those with intellectual disabilities have been left vulnerable from the US values of independence and competition. For this reason, parents of children with intellectual disabilities have arguably found it harder under this model. In England, while the extension of rights towards disabled people has not stretched as far, the reliance on the welfare state and community support for adults with intellectual disabilities has arguably better served carers. However, as an attempt to support disabled people and their families in the community, the English welfare state still remains a contradiction; 'it has produced both benefits and problems, it has included and excluded, it will empower and it will disempower' (Oliver and Barnes, 1998: 5). For the most part however, while such policies do not go as far as empowering carers, the English landscape of care supports them more attentively in their daily lives.

Ireland by contrast, has developed very differently to both these countries. It thus serves as an interesting and timely case-study in these broad welfare debates. Firstly, Ireland did not share the same levels of wealth that existed in either nation until late in the 20th century. Secondly, the role of the nonprofit sector, which originally comprised the Catholic Church, became the dominant provider of welfare. In the Irish case, women's role in the family was held by the Church and State as the cornerstone of society, thus having later consequences for carers. The insights learned from this comparative perspective offer important lessons for other jurisdictions, where proponents of welfare reform in England and US are arguing for a move away from state 'welfare' models towards 'bottom-up' grass-roots approaches (Power and Kenny, in press).

This chapter details the progression of caring in Ireland from its unparalleled institutional regime to its 'relaxed-control' community care model by examining the policies that made it happen. Over the last two centuries, significant changes have taken place in the way people with intellectual disabilities and their families have been treated in Ireland. This chapter traces Ireland's efforts at creating its own range of social rights and services for carers (see timeline in Table 6.1).

The Early Development of Asylums

During the 18th and 19th centuries, Ireland shared much of the same legislative history concerning the 'care' of those with intellectual disabilities and their families as England through the implementation of the British Acts, although there were many additional Acts made specifically for Ireland. Furthermore, the British influence continued long after independence as the proximity of Britain inevitably meant that comparisons have and continue to be made between the social services in the two countries (Curry, 1998).

According to Robert's (2001) timeline, which traces the history of legislation relating to people with intellectual disabilities, the social setting in Ireland provided an atypical developmental arena for asylums, particularly with such factors as

Table 6.1 Irish Disability and Care Legislation

Discourse	Legislation	Purpose of Legislation
1226–1707 English Statutes		
Promotion of punitive view of dependency and disability.	*1601 Poor Law Act*	Established indoor relief in almshouses and outdoor relief, where poor were left in their own homes and would be given either a 'dole' of money on which to live or be given relief in kind – clothes and food.
1707–1800 Pre-Union British Statutes		
Made the first distinction between paupers and lunatics.	*1744 Vagrancy Act*	Made some provision for the treatment of care of lunatics from parish relief funds. This saw the growth of privately owned institutions across the country known as 'madhouses'.
1800 Union with Ireland Act		
Promotion of Institutional Care.	*1817 Irish Lunatic Asylums for the Poor Act*	Legislative provision of public asylums for the entire country.
	1821 Irish Lunatic Asylums for the Poor Act	Formed the basis of the existing code of laws which provided for the formation of asylum districts. An Act to make more effectual Provision for the Establishment of Asylums for the Lunatic Poor, and for the Custody of Insane Persons charged with Offences in Ireland.
	1825 Irish Lunatic Asylums Act	England consolidated and amended the Laws relating to institutions in Ireland.
	1825 Local Government Act	Provided for the substitution of the term 'district mental hospital' for the term 'district lunatic asylum'.
	1828 Madhouse Act	Established a stricter regime of licensing and visiting committees for asylums.
	1838 Poor Relief (Ireland) Act	Introduced a means-tested adaptation of the English Poor Law 1838.
	1842 Private Lunatic Asylums (Ireland) Act	Introduced legal control over private institutions. Provided for the inspection of private institutions, the regulation of their management and the admission of patients thereto. Institutions other than charitable institutions supported wholly or in part by voluntary contributions and not kept for profit by any private individual were required to be licensed annually by the Quarter Sessions Courts.
	1845 Lunacy (Ireland) Act	Made two important provisions – for the removal of all lunatics from the houses of industry to the district lunatic asylums and it gave power for the establishment of an asylum for chronic or harmless patients for each of the provinces. No steps were taken to implement this latter provision.

Table 6.1 continued

Discourse	Legislation	Purpose of Legislation
continued	*1867 Lunacy (Ireland) Act*	Empowered any two justices of the peace to commit to the district lunatic asylum any person apprehended or discovered under circumstances denoting derangement of mind and a purpose of committing an indictable crime.
	1898 Local Government (Ireland) Act	Substituted a power enabling asylum authorities to establish auxiliary asylums for the reception of patients who, being chronic lunatics, were not dangerous to themselves or others and were medically certified not to require special care and treatment in a fully equipped lunatic asylum.
	1898 Vagrancy Act.	Amended and extended English Vagrancy Act to Ireland.
	1901 Lunacy (Ireland) Act.	Established that a person had to be received into a district mental hospital deemed to be a criminal lunatic.
Assumption of a male breadwinner supporting his dependent wife and children.	*1911 National Insurance Act*	Introduced the first social insurance scheme.
	1913 National Insurance Act.	Made provision for compulsory insurance against unemployment in the 'insured trades'.
	1913 Mental Deficiency Act	Extended the English Mental Deficiency Act to Ireland.
Acknowledgement of need for disability insurance.	*1920 National Health Insurance Act*	Established a combined compulsory health and disability insurance.
Irish Statutes		
Catholic Church teachings dominant. Advocated minimal role for the state.	*1921–1929 National Health Insurance Acts 1933–1934 National Health Insurance Acts*	Incremental amendments to health and disability insurance.
	1934 Public Assistance Act	Provided assistance to a poor person who was unable to provide by his own industry or other lawful means the medical, surgical or dental treatment, or medicines, or medical, surgical or dental appliances necessary for himself or any persons whom he is liable under this Act to maintain shall be eligible for medical assistance.

Need to reform asylum care rather than replace it.	*1945 Mental Treatment Act*	The first signs of Irish reform of the asylum system of care.
	1948 Social Welfare (Reciprocal Arrangements) Act	Established comprehensive social security plan to provide insurance against old age, illness, blindness.
Acknowledgement of need for greater statutory role in healthcare.	*1953 Health Act*	Changed the role of the state in relation to health care – it was now extended beyond prevention to include the organisation and financing of curative medicine for wide groups of the population. Also marked the beginning of a change in the relationship between statutory and voluntary sectors with the Section 65 grants for non-profit organisations providing services 'similar or ancillary' to their own.
Idea of institutionalisation persisted.	*1953 Mental Treatment Act*	Amended and extended the Mental Treatment Act, 1945. Entitled a person in charge of approved institutions in which it is desired to have such person received and detained and his officers, assistants, and servants and any medical officer of such institution to receive and take charge of a person. With a medical certificate.
	1954 Health Act	Amended and extended the Health Act, 1947.
	1957 Voluntary Health Insurance (VHI) Act	Established the voluntary insurance scheme in Ireland.
	1952 Social Welfare Act	Made limited changes to the Norton bill, so that it became a less extensive version. In the end however Fianna Fáil abandoned Dr Ryan's plan, cut back Norton's proposals and implemented what was left.
	1960–1968 Social Welfare Acts	Incremental amendments to health and disability payments.
First realisation of burden on full-time carers.	*1969 Social Welfare Act*	Established the Prescribed Relative's Allowance. It was initially confined to cases where a qualified pensioner was being cared for on a full-time basis by a daughter or step-daughter who gave up long-standing employment in order to provide that care.
Acknowledgement of the need for a more modern health care service.	*1970 Health Act*	Principal Act governing health care in Ireland. Set up the Health Board regional structure.
Acknowledgement of work provided by women carers.	*1989 Social Welfare Act*	Paid the Prescribed Relative's Allowance directly to the carer, however it remained very restrictive and very small financially.

Table 6.1 continued

Discourse	Legislation	Purpose of Legislation
continued	*1990 Social Welfare Act*	Introduced a means-tested 'Carer's Allowance' (CA), a social assistance payment payable to someone who resides with or has a direct link with, and provides full-time care to a person who is so incapacitated as to require full-time care.
	1996 Health (Amendment) Act	Brought new obligations and opportunities for the Health Boards, to work collectively in pursuit of the strategic objectives as set out in the government's health strategy. It became apparent at an early stage, that a formal structure was required to facilitate this collective working and which would in particular establish a framework.
Recognised need to educate disabled children in less-segregated settings.	*1998 Education Act*	Required recognised schools (in effect those funded by the State) to use their available resources to ensure that the education needs of all students, including those with a disability, are identified and provided for.
	1999 Health (Eastern Regional Health Authority) Act	Established three Area Health Boards and an Eastern Regional Health Authority which will oversee the operation of those boards.
	1999 National Disability Act	Set up the National Disability Authority.
	1999 Social Welfare Act	Established the Respite Care Grant of £200, or such higher amount as may be prescribed, to be paid to a relevant carer each year in respect of the cost of respite care.
Recognised disability as a possible ground for discrimination.	*2000 Equal Status Act*	Prohibited the discrimination in relation to the supply of goods, facilities and services on nine grounds including disability.
Greater recognition of carers' burden in society.	*2001 Carer's Leave Act*	Introduced Carer's Benefit to make it possible for workers to take a temporary leave of 18 months to become a carer without loss of employment.
	2004 Health Act	Established the Health Service Executive to replace the regional Health Boards. Introduced January 2005.

colonisation, the lack of a classic pattern of industrialisation, and a population which had severe periods of rapid decline coupled with chronic and enduring emigration (Brennan, 2004: 498). After the *Act of Union* 1800, the British Imperial government made numerous but unsuccessful attempts to address the extreme and widespread poverty in Ireland. No simple model of exploitation can be applied to what was an exceedingly complex economic relationship between the two islands. Ireland was not consistently the victim of a crude, economic imperialism; however at particular times, and within particular areas of the relationship, the evidence for exploitation is more persuasive (Kenny, 2004). The Poorhouse was an unpopular and unsuitable location for 'idiots' or 'feeble-minded' people. However since the notion of treating madness or mental handicap did not yet exist, the managers of the hospitals and workhouses, where many insane and 'feeble-minded' people found themselves, subdued their behaviour by any means necessary.

The 'care' of Irish 'idiots' and 'insane' came under the direct control of the Lord Lieutenant. The rhetoric of asylum, taking place in England and across western Europe, ended up finding a piece of testing ground in Ireland, where the Lord Lieutenant's office had the freedom to enact legislation with little resistance. The *Report of the Select Committee to Consider the State of the Lunatic Poor in Ireland* (1817) led to Ireland becoming the first nation in the world to pass legislation, the *Irish Lunatic Asylums for the Poor Act* (1817), requiring the development of a national framework of publicly funded asylums. This came long before its English counterpart. According to Finnane (1981), 'what England saw only in 1845, Ireland had already witnessed in essentials in 1817: the legislative provision of public asylums for the entire country' (cited in Roberts, 2001).

This national publicly-funded infrastructure of institutions both consumed and generated large amounts of finance and was a major source of employment in many large towns (Brennan, 2004). It was the first national bureaucratic system established through colonial social policy, occurring 17 years earlier than the development of the Irish national school system in 1834 (Brennan, 2004). By the time England had established its own asylum system in 1845 (and the US established its first asylum, the Massachusetts School for the Idiotic and Feeble-minded, in 1849), the rate of admissions to Irish institutions was far greater than that experienced in both these countries (World Health Organisation, 1961). The context at the time during the mid-nineteenth century was characterised by an uneasy political climate, and the acceptance by the public of the 1817 Act, a deeply flawed law (Prior, 2003). Since England's colonisation of Ireland, asylums were seen as an essential guarantor of the social order (Heller, 1997).

Alongside the institutions, many people with intellectual disabilities were never incarcerated but cared for in the family home 'in the shadow of the asylum'. Services for families looking after people with disabilities at home were largely nonexistent. Furthermore, people had to deal with the notion of intellectual disability as the stigmatised source of perceived hereditary problems, which later became a powerful discourse by the medical profession. In cases where someone was cared for at home, there was a degree of embarrassment within households.

On the face of it, families did not have much control over the lives of their child, although on occasion were able to get the better of the authorities who preferred to institutionalise the child rather than let them be brought up at home (Thomson, 1996). At this time, the idea of 'informal carers' was unheard of.

Following from this, the *Irish Lunatic Asylums for the Poor Act* (1821) was to make more effective provision for the establishment of asylums for the 'lunatic and mentally handicapped poor', and for the custody of insane persons charged with offences in Ireland. Most people with an intellectual disability who were not living at home were therefore cared for under this legislation, primarily in the poorhouse or the insane asylum (Robins, 1992: 29). In 1825 England consolidated and amended the Laws relating to institutions in Ireland; Section 55[1] provided that the Inspector General of Prisons should visit and inspect (amongst other places) every madhouse and place where lunatics or idiots were confined (Roberts, 2001). This reflected the way in which expertise and authority in disability related matters was envisioned.

The *Lunatics Act* (1845) established the asylum system as the proper and primary system for the treatment of lunacy and idiocy. This made it compulsory for each county to provide an asylum within three years of its passing. Prior to this legislation, asylums had differed markedly in size and quality of care. Many different explanations have been cited for the development of this elaborate system of asylum care. Firstly, it is seen to have been a result of the spread of Enlightenment thinking, where the application of scientific reason could offer solutions to society's problems and difficulties. Secondly, it is argued that the rise of industrialisation which led to the transition from agriculture and cottage-based industries to 'waged-based' systems demarcated disabled people as less-productive (Gleeson, 1999). However, in Ireland, this was less-clear, as agriculture and cottage-based industries were still common throughout the 19th century. What was more evident in the Irish case was the entrusting faith in institutions as a balm to disordered minds and a critical tool for rehabilitation:

> The provision of a suitable building is in fact a most essential condition to any judicious form of treatment. The treatment of the lunatic is to by accomplished not merely *in* but *by* the Asylum, which may be looked upon as a great therapeutic instrument itself, without which the efforts of the physicians could accomplish little (Fogerty, 1867)

This resonates with Philo's work (1987) which drew attention to the way people with disabilities were 'cared for', in particular, mental patients in England. Thus the nineteenth-century asylum, as understood by writers such as William Fogerty, was both logically and self-consciously designed by concerned, paternal agencies as an elaborate map or model to guide lunatics.

---

1 Of 'An Act for consolidating and amending the Laws relating to Prisons in Ireland'.

At the turn of the mid-nineteenth-century, the Irish famine followed on the heels of the Irish Poor Law. This contributed to a social context in which certain members of society, including the unemployed, the old and the disabled, existed in a position of vulnerability and uncertainty. In the absence of resources within the family and community that could support these people in the community, it was inevitable that people with intellectual disabilities would end up institutionalised (Brennan, 2004). In the lunatic asylums, the steady rise in admissions continued, with the ten existing district insane asylums now overcrowded and inadequate. Despite this, the curative emphasis of asylums was still being heralded by the medical profession. According to Dr Nugent in his 'Observations on the Report of the Commissioners of Inquiry into Lunatic Asylums (Ireland) (Nugent, 1958), '[institutions] were eminently successful as curative establishments…a wondrous immunity…from accidents and deeds of violence, considering the excitability of our race'. In reality, the institutions quickly degraded due to over population, under-funding, and mismanagement. During the 1850s and 1860s, the authorities embarked upon the development of 12 additional asylums as well as expanding those already existing (Torrey and Miller, 2007). The great expansion of the Irish asylum system was thus clearly being influenced by the economic factors associated with the famine, and a way to deal with the associated changes in the structure of family life.

As with Britain, the *Idiots Act* (1886), and the *Lunacy Act* (1890) were also applied to Ireland. The *Idiots Act* required that authorities establish asylums for the care, education and training of the 'idiots'. Administrating control was only valid if a medical 'expert' was in charge. Much of the early psychological profession however believed that madness and idiocy were actually caused by defective and/or careless families, thus leading to their proper 'moral treatment' in asylums (Jones, 2002). It allowed rates to be raised for building a 'mental deficiency colony'. It also required the registration and inspection of the institutions and hospitals (Warren, 2003). The *Lunacy Act* defined lunatic as 'an idiot or person of unsound mind" and enshrined involuntary incarceration which led to even more extensive institutionalisation in Ireland than in Britain (Robins, 1986). Young men in particular who had profound intellectual disabilities were more likely to be admitted than women, because they were regarded as more difficult to control at home.

At the turn of the century, the *Lunacy (Ireland) Act* (1901) was seen as copper fastening this custodial approach and consolidated much previous legislation. The medical takeover of matters concerning social conformity in lunacy and mental handicap was also experienced in Ireland at the turn of the 20th century. Doctors were successful in harnessing the collective power of their profession to gain occupational status and security within the Irish asylum system. However, the discourse of eugenics was not as pervasive in Ireland at the end of the 19th century, with the national colonisation of the country being a more dominant narrative in debates over the disfavoured British models of care being enforced (Finnane, 1981).

It was not until the early 20th century that any type of special provision for those with intellectual disability was made available in Ireland and this came in the form of the *Mental Deficiency Act* (1913). Like England, this led to a very rudimentary system of 'community care'. The Act defined four classes of defective – idiots, imbeciles, feeble-minded persons and moral defectives. It established the Board of Control which took over the powers of the Lunacy Commission; provided for mental defectives to be sent to institutions or be placed under guardianship; and made the care and supervision of mental defectives the responsibility of County and County Borough Councils. In the early period after Ireland established the Free State, the British Royal Commission on Lunacy and Mental Disorder (1926) had recommended a community service instead of detention for the 'feeble minded' based on the treatment of patients in their own homes wherever possible (Warren, 2003). From the period of independence however, Ireland developed their own separate policy from England on the care of those with intellectual disabilities and their families.

Irish Partition (1922–1944)

After the establishment of the Free State (1922), there was little development in social welfare for people with intellectual disabilities or their families. The Irish welfare system, having inherited the Poor Law, catered exclusively for the poor. The early 1920s saw the abolition of Poor Law unions across Ireland (with the initial exception of Dublin) and the closure of workhouses to reduce costs (National Archives of Ireland, 2004). Unfortunately, in the early period after Ireland established the Free State, the *British Royal Commission on Lunacy and Mental Disorder* (1926) had recommended a community service instead of detention for the 'mentally retarded' based on the treatment of patients in their own homes wherever possible (Warren, 2003). From the period of independence however, Ireland developed their own separate policy from England on the care of those with intellectual disabilities and their families.

The Irish State on its foundation was influenced by the specific social class and gender construction of Irish society and by ideological factors, in particular, the role of the Roman Catholic Church (the Church). In 1929, for example, the government reinforced the male breadwinner assumption of women's dependency by providing that a woman's membership of the insurance scheme terminated on marriage (McLaughlin, 1993). It was clear that the State was reliant on the Church for both political support and for welfare and education provision. A 1931 Papal Encyclical[2] *Quadragesimo Anno* espoused the principle of 'subsidiarity' as a means of circumscribing state encroachment on voluntary welfare and charity arrangements within the parish or local community (Grogan, 1978). This principle was broadly accepted by government, which meant the state would have a

2 Letter from the Pope to the Irish Bishops.

functional role of ensuring social order, however, it would refrain from intervening in economic and social affairs unless the national interest or social equilibrium was threatened. The Encyclical stated that: 'It is an injustice and at the same time a great evil and disturbance of right order to assign to a greater and higher association what lesser and subordinate organisations can do'. The Church was able to capitalise upon the aspirations for Irish nationhood due to the high rates of Roman Catholic followers. According to McLaughlin (1993) the Church provided the institutional links between the new political, economic and social elites and the masses. The religious-based organisations tended to emphasise charitable principles and the duty of the rich to help the needy. People with disabilities and their families had to therefore depend on being supported by ad hoc voluntary groups and under-funded charities. With high mortality rates more generally, due to heart disease, tuberculosis and cancer, very few people with intellectual disabilities lived until adulthood (Muckross Research Library, no date).

As a consequence of the Church's dominant position, according to Inglis 'secular civility became synonymous with Catholic morality' (1987: 165). This culminated in notions of Catholic teachings being enshrined in Article 41.2 of the 1937 Constitution, a document drawn up by both the government of the time (Fianna Fáil) and the Church in which the family was recognised as the 'natural, primary, and fundamental unit of Society…indispensable to the welfare of the Nation and the State'. The role of women was institutionally confined to the home:

> the State recognises that by her life with the home, woman gives to the State a support without which the common good cannot be achieved. The State shall, therefore, endeavour to ensure that mothers shall not be obliged by necessity to engage in labour to the neglect of their duties in the home (Article 41.2, 1937 Constitution)

Surprisingly, all political parties broadly shared this view and, unlike in the UK, there was little public debate about an alternative approach. The Church's strength in shaping historical discourses in how care is arranged appears to have left a legacy on how care support is arranged today. Ireland's early social welfare policies were thus very gendered, as women were seen as part of a broader family unit and as economically dependent on men, while men were considered the provider. de Valera, the Irish Taoiseach[3] argued that, 'our aim ought to be that the breadwinner, who is normally and naturally in these cases, when alive, the father of the family, should be able by his work to bring in enough to maintain the whole household' (McLaughlin, 1993: 211). Fianna Fáil remained fiscally conservative in its outlook and maintained its policy mix of protectionism, industrial development, agricultural policy and limited welfare measures. No coherent Keynesian approach appeared in Irish economic policy until much later than in England or the US.

---

3 Prime Minister of the Government of Ireland.

Women's groups fought against the 'sinister and retrogressive' provisions of the constitution (McLaughlin, 1993). In the late 1930s Muintir na Tíre[4] became an important mobilising force for local communities, spurring women on to greater voluntary activity and constantly emphasising the theme of growth through self reliance. Women were denied access to legal aid and no welfare was available as of right to unmarried mothers or deserted wives. Women were also refused the right to inherit land. Therefore women who were involved in caring duties in the home had limited rights and entitlements, which were only available to the husband. Furthermore the principle of subsidiarity meant that neither the state nor the Church provided a system of support for families of children with intellectual disabilities apart from the inherited Victorian institutions.

At this time, the social welfare system as we know it today simply did not exist. The administration of the social welfare system was the responsibility of a range of different departments including the Department of Local Government, Industry and Commerce, and the Revenue Commissioners (Cousins, 1995: 19). Some steps were made to try and co-ordinate the system, with the establishment of the National Health Insurance Society (NHIS) in 1935 to amalgamate all individual insurance societies to increase benefits and decrease the cost of running national health insurance. A Catholic Bishop, Dr John Dignan was appointed as the first chairman (Barrington, 1987). However the late 1930s and early 1940s saw very little movement in social policy, apart from a children's allowance introduced in 1944 (Daly and Clavero, 2003).

Catholic State (1945–1959)

In the beginning of the post-World War Two period (1945–54) several Irish responses to the UK Beveridge report were published including proposals for the expansion of the Irish system. One major difference however, was that Ireland did not share in the same economic prosperity experienced in Britain or the US in the post-war period. Around the time when Britain was setting up the NHS and the welfare state, the Irish State's inability to afford such welfare provision appeared even starker.

Given the role of the Church in the formation of the State, Ireland also had a weak civil society, except for rural Meitheal[5] schemes and the Society of St Vincent de Paul. Friendly Societies in Ireland had a very limited and dispersed coverage which meant the national-insurance system could not utilise them to administer social welfare, like they did in the UK. This weak civil society had further implications in 1946 when there was no formal public consultation in relation to the drafting of the Irish White Paper on Social Welfare, in contrast to Beveridge, who had received evidence from about 130 organisations, representing a very wide range of interests

---

4 The national organisation promoting community development in Ireland.

5 Meitheal was an Irish term for farming solidarity and voluntary work-sharing schemes.

(Cousins, 1995: 184–6). This weakness in Irish civil society meant the State only had the Church to look for help in its decision-making.

Although the Church played a more primary role in social policy areas such as education and health, it also made concerted efforts to influence the social welfare system. One of the main Irish responses to the Beveridge Report was an article published by a prominent Catholic theologian and future bishop Rev. Cornelius Lucey, who did not support its application in Ireland. Instead he advocated the retention of a (modified) means-tested system, the introduction of pay-related contributions and benefits, and the administration of the scheme by a vocational body such as the NHIS (Cousins, 1995: 18). The Church remained wary of state intervention and encroachment in welfare matters, stressing that it would undermine the voluntary sector, resulting in higher taxation and violating Catholic social teaching and the opportunity of practising Christian charity (McLaughlin, 1993). This meant social services were underdeveloped in Ireland. The Church saw any secular involvement such as social workers in families as the state being intrusive. The Catholic Church was concerned about what they saw as 'the evils of socialism' and was perhaps somewhat dubious about the scientific study of social problems. The Catholic Church made it quite clear that social action should be Church-led. This was quite distinct from the (Protestant) Church of Ireland, which saw social service as chiefly the responsibility of laymen (Kearney and Skehill, 2005).

In the June 1944 election, Irish public opinion sought social services on a par with those available in Northern Ireland. Fianna Fáil was forced to put much more emphasis on social policy measures than before. They established a Cabinet Committee to examine and report on a new Department of Social Services (Barrington, 1987). At the same time, the chairman of the NHIS, Bishop Dr John Dignan also published proposals for reform of social security. However, this caused a major political dispute, as Seán MacEntee (then Minister for Local Government) took extreme exception to the fact that the bishop had published his proposals rather than presenting them to himself and his department in the first case (Cousins, 1995). Dignan proposed major reforms of both the existing health and social security services. It was highly critical of existing services, describing them as still tainted with pauperism and destitution. His plan received very widespread support from a broad range of political parties, trade unions, and other organisations. However MacEntee remained opposed and stated that the bishop's proposals were entirely impracticable, indicating a very strained working relationship between the NHIS and the Department. However the public quarrel increased pressure on the government to produce some alternative response (Cousins, 1995).

As a result of the rudimentary welfare service planning, fundamental issues relating to the delivery of Irish disability services were not well addressed. Although the earlier legislation in England applied, the first sign of Irish reform of the asylum system of care was the 1945 *Mental Treatment Act*. This stated that the Inspector of Mental Hospitals was required to inspect every mental hospital in the country once a year. If the hospital was being run privately, the Inspector was required to inspect it twice a year. However, as we shall discover in the following time period, these reports were routinely ignored. Moreover, the Act still allowed for having a person committed involuntarily. The year the Act was passed, it was clear that the problem of the increasing numbers of involuntary psychiatric inpatients was reaching crisis level. One of the aims of Ireland's *Mental Treatment Act* (1945) was to reduce the numbers of persons in asylums. There were some 17,708 individuals resident in asylums in the Republic of Ireland during this time (Walsh and Daly, 2004). Institutions had become huge isolated, self-sufficient places, segregated spaces and significant economic spaces in Ireland. St Davnet's Hospital for example, had almost 900 inpatients and St Ita's on Lambay Island had over 2,000 inmates. The sheer size of these institutions led to much stigma for those who were being treated within them. The damage for people with intellectual disabilities was largely related to the loss of an individual identity and the complete segregation from one's former life, including family, work and community.

The pressure to co-ordinate services culminated in 1947 with the establishment of a unified Department of Social Welfare, under the new Minister, William Norton, which took over responsibility for the majority of social welfare schemes. This successfully merged the NHIS with the Department. As well as the administrative logic for its establishment, one of the key reasons for its creation was the growing anticipation from government and the public of further developments in social welfare services. With the growth that was happening abroad, it was a period where the modernisation of the State's role was greatly envisaged (Cousins, 1995). A further question mark existed over whether or not to amalgamate health and social welfare services in one department. However many administrative and inter-departmental battles constrained any real interest in incorporating both. The Department of Health was formally established as a department on its own in 1947 (Disability Federation of Ireland, 2002).

The *Health Act* (1953) marked the beginning of a change in the relationship between statutory and voluntary sectors with the introduction of Section 65 grants for non-profit organisations.[6] This allowed health authorities to support voluntary organisations providing services 'similar or ancillary' to their own. An exact definition of 'similar' or 'ancillary' was not laid down in legislation; neither were they defined by the courts. This funding model provided global grants directly to the agencies on the basis of the previous year's financial outturn, proposals to improve or expand services, and the availability of finance generally (Ryan, 1999). As long as the outcomes that were originally proposed by the service provider were delivered in the end, there was little transparency on what money was being spent on what resources. Issues such as staff costs, transport costs and care costs remained opaque. Moreover, there was typically little connection between the size of the grant and the numbers cared for, the

---

6 The independent sector of disability providers in Ireland is solely comprised of non-profit organisations. The private sector has never developed within the Irish disability service provider landscape.

category or the degree of disability (C&AG, 2005). The funding has since been discretionary, a fact which has been much criticised. In addition, there was considerable differences between health service areas in the interpretation of this section. A focal point of argument in the past was the lack of a definition of a particular set of 'core services'. O'Sullivan remarks that the development of 'core services' would have implied the establishment of clear criteria for their provision and eligibility and the provision of ear-marked funding for them (Disability Federation of Ireland, 2002).

In the period 1950–59, it was clear that Ireland's economic management left a lot to be desired. National income expanded at less that 1 per cent per annum and industrial employment actually fell by 14 per cent in this period (McLaughlin, 1993: 213). While Fianna Fáil's ideology had been associated with de Valera's vision of an independent, Catholic Ireland, the party had to modernise its role in economic and social policy. While it retained its reliance on clientalist strategies, which meant that at the local level, individuals went to their local politicians seeking remedy for their specific problems, it positioned itself as a centre right party. By the end of the decade, Ireland became an export-oriented economy. Irish people became more liberal and outward looking. MacEntee (Minister for Health) made no major overhaul of the health service and was intent on just 'oiling the machine'. Barrington (1987) commented that the combined effect of the *Health Act* (1953) and the *Voluntary Health Insurance Act* (1957), which introduced voluntary insurance, resulted in the ordinary Irish people benefiting from a health service of an incomparably higher standard than in the 1940s.

The number of in-patients in public psychiatric hospitals in Ireland in 1958 however was at an all time high of 21,075 (Daly and Walsh, 2002). While this period was characterised by major structural reforms of health and social services, there was still little or no statutory role in the provision of community care services for family carers. The state appeared quite content to operate almost at arm's length with regard to many social services and were beginning to look at ways of offloading the inherited Victorian institutions. The department began to look to the Church for ways to expand the mental handicap services. The state was focused on getting Ireland back on track, and church motivations were to underpin religious objectives. To a large extent, disability policy was left to the sidelines and entrenched in the ideology of institutions. In terms of methods for providing accommodation for people with intellectual disabilities, institutions run wholly by religious orders were ranked first. Dr Vincent J. Dolphin was appointed Inspector of Mental Hospitals in 1953. He was instructed to 'get in touch with various religious orders in the country with a view to expanding whatever service was already provided' (Ryan, 1999). This would have been suitable if this expansion of service was to form part of a fully comprehensive service designed to work in tandem with the statutory bodies, but this is not what happened. With considerable grants of land and buildings made to Religious Orders, the *entire* service for people with intellectual disabilities was ceded to a few religious orders. Meanwhile, professional social work for families was constrained by the Catholic hegemony.

Welfare Expansion (1960–1969)

Throughout the 1960s, Ireland tried to lift itself to a level close to the other, richer European countries with Sean Lemass leading the way for the modernisation of Irish society. However, Ireland missed out on the first period of economic prosperity experienced by Western countries in the early 1960s and suffered enormous rates of emigration. The depth of the economic crisis resulted in a radical rethink of the Irish state's involvement in the economy (McLaughlin, 1993). Economic planning was adopted as part of a modernisation strategy and free trade was embraced. The Irish Development Authority (IDA) was given the responsibility to secure the location of multi-national corporations in Ireland. Through a generous tax package and administering the world's first free-trade zone, a major inflow of foreign investment occurred. This period saw an upturn in the Irish economy with international investment.

Although there was an expansion of the welfare state, it showed very little signs of crossing over class boundaries. Instead, manual workers had to carry the burden of paying social insurance, while those in the higher classes were considered less exposed to insurable risks. According to Cousins, it 'was accomplished in such a manner as to leave privilege essentially undisturbed' (Cousins, 1995). Although the Church gave its blessing to state efforts to resolve economic problems by applying modified neo-liberal economic principles, it was less prepared to condone any liberalisation of state policies which it viewed as threatening family life (Hannigan, 1990, cited in McLaughlin, 1993: 225).

At the time, 'mental handicap' was still a taboo subject with the mainstream public knowing little about it. The rate of institutionalisation of people with mental illness and intellectual disabilities was still high. According to Census statistics from the Medico-Social Research Board/Health Research Board, there were 19,801 psychiatric in-patients in 1963. This consisted of people diagnosed with Schizophrenia, a mental disability, dementia, and a large number who were unspecified (Daly and Walsh, May 2002). The WHO produced a report in 1961 which rated Ireland highest in the world in the number of beds in residential institutions (10.8 per 1,000 total population). This was largely to do with the unavailability of informal/family care due to Ireland's traditionally low marriage rate, which was a result of Irish patterns of farm inheritance in rural areas. This was based on an inheritance system which allowed for the transfer of undivided land tenure from generation to generation – that is, it only permitted the marriage of those men who would inherit the family land (one in each family) and those women who would become their wives (Salazar, 2003). The price to be paid for the correct working of this system was a low marriage rate, as well as weak caregiver networks and a high rate of institutionalisation.

Around this time there was increased pressure to de-institutionalise and move to community care which came from increased international concerns for civil rights. The Government White Paper: *The Problem of the Mentally Handicapped* (1960) recognised considerable difficulty in providing services for 'mentally handicapped' due to a disparity of view as to whose responsibility the provision of services was. The White Paper indicated this disparity yet could not agree whether services should be provided by the Department of Health, Education, or Social Welfare. The Department of Health favoured an extension of the activities by the Church. Significantly, it was at this time, that all the hospitals were renamed with saints' names. For example, an overflow of Richmond Asylum was built and called St Ita's; Grangegorman was changed to St Brendan's; Ballinasloe to St Brigid's; and Mullingar to St Loman's.

The state also started to fund some smaller lay charity and voluntary organisations. A co-ordinating body, called NAMHI, the National Association for the Mentally Handicapped of Ireland (since renamed Inclusion Ireland) was founded in 1961, and has since become the co-ordinating body for over 160 organisations providing services and support to almost 28,000 people with intellectual disabilities in Ireland. It has since provided a central forum for its members to identify priorities and formulate nationally agreed policies to present to government, statutory bodies, other relevant groups as well as the general public (NAMHI, 2004).

In 1961, a *Commission of Inquiry on Mental Handicap* was appointed to examine and report on the arrangements for the care of 'mentally handicapped'. It took the Commission an impressively long time span of five years to produce a report, in the mean time allowing government to halt any progress or future developments. Although the report marked a watershed in the development of community-based services in Ireland, it mirrored *The Problem of the Mentally Handicapped* White Paper, in terms of noting the preferability of providing these services through religious orders and voluntary bodies (Robins, 1992: 55). This policy decision had a considerable impact on Irish service provision to the present day (Quin and Redmond, 2005). Despite the increased emphasis on the importance of community care, expenditure patterns did not reflect any noticeable shift, towards community care services as opposed to hospital services. The Irish reform of institutions remained at best aspirational. Unfortunately, families who got placements for their sons or daughters in these institutions were considered the lucky ones; the other bleak choice for families was to 'get on with it' as best they could (Ryan, 1999). Little did they know the shocking conditions in many of the hospitals, where lighting, ventilation, sanitary and culinary conditions were abject, as discovered by the Assistant Inspector for Mental Hospitals (Ramsay, 1958).

The further growth of voluntary organisations tried to address gaps in state service provision (Quin, 2005: 153). Some of these organisations grew very large over time and began to employ a wide range of personnel. These included Brothers of Charity Services and 'Muiriosa' (The Sisters of Charity of Jesus and Mary). The provision of professional community-based services such as social work, physiotherapy, and many educational and training services was by voluntary rather than statutory services. There was also a significant increase in 'lay' Parent and Friends Associations which grew organically in various parts of the country. This was in response to the bleak choice for families to 'get on with it' as best they could, or to place their child on a waiting list for residential services: families in desperate circumstances expected to give up their child. While government endlessly deliberated and continuously talked of extensions to existing institutions, parents of children with intellectual disabilities were becoming very active across the country at setting up local voluntary services.

One parent, Patsy Farrell, for example, was aware of the great lack of services to meet the needs of her son. She placed a letter in the personal column of The Irish Times and in other papers, asking parents in the Dublin area to get in touch with her about starting a day school for children with intellectual disabilities. Following a more positive response than expected, St Michael's House was established. The organisation provided the first day service in Ireland. A second St Michael's House day centre opened in Grosvenor Road and the service has continued growing ever since. Other examples began to take place around the country and many parents and friends associations became significant providers of supports to family carers of young adults with intellectual disabilities.

The first sign of acknowledging the need for supporting long-term care of an adult in the home was the 'Constant Attendance Allowance'. This was introduced in 1967 under the occupational injuries scheme and was payable to a person who, as a result of an occupational accident or disease, was suffering from 100 per cent disablement and who required constant attendance. However, because it required such an exceptional level of disablement, the rate of carers in receipt of the payment was low. It thus contained an efficient method of cost containment.

Shortly after establishing this rudimentary payment, the government also introduced the 'Prescribed Relative's Allowance' in 1969, a form of recompense to a daughter or other prescribed relative who would look after elderly parents in their homes rather than have them looked after in institutions. It was introduced for people then over 70 years of age who were severely incapacitated. According to McLaughlin (1994: 276), Ireland thus became one of the first Western European countries to introduce a financial payment for informal care, due to concern about the high levels of residential care among the elderly population. The origins of the benefit suggest that it was primarily intended to discourage institutionalisation rather than to provide income maintenance for informal/family carers directly (McLaughlin, 1994: 276). It came in the form of an increased pension, however in practice, it was only daughters or stepdaughters who could avail of it, not the person's spouse. It was thus very restrictive and reflected the expected gender role in society at the time. By 1972, the scheme extended to male relatives and social welfare contributions were credited to those who gave up employment to provide care (O'Louglin, 2005). However, the rate of institutionalisation only started declining in the 1980s at a very slow rate.

At the other end of the life cycle was the 'Domiciliary Care Allowance' which has since been paid to the parents of children with disabilities and is not means-tested on the parent's income. A child must be under the age of 16, and must have a severe disability that is likely to last for at least one year. In practice then, the recipient must need substantially more constant care and attention than a child of the same age who does not have a disability. There have been no rigid medical guidelines, regarding the type of disability a qualifying child must have. Instead it is a matter for the Senior Area Medical Officer in the health board to determine whether a child with a particular condition qualifies for the Allowance (Welfare.ie, 2004).

These benefits demonstrated that the state began to offer some recompense to the work of women in Irish society. Developments such as the Women's and Trade Union Movements and the *National Commission on the Status of Women* (1969) proved very influential in the development of the ideology of empowerment, participation, social inclusion and voluntary action. It condemned the extent of the discriminatory treatment of Irish women (Brennan, 1979). From this time, campaigning and advocacy became increasingly important in the disability area (McCarron, 1991). This led to an increase in the number of women setting up their own associations and lay services. Furthermore, in combination with the emergence of the Irish women's movement and the help of the EC, these changes led to a slight weakening of the Church's position

Health Act and Beginnings of Community Care (1970–1979)

In 1970, Fianna Fáil brought in the *Health Act* (1970), which was deemed the principal Act governing health care for the next 30 years in Ireland (Disability Federation of Ireland, 2002). It set up the Irish Health Board structure (with eight health boards) to provide health services around the country. Up until this point, there were 27 unified health authorities within the 4 most populated counties (Curry, 1998). The reasons behind it were that the state had taken over the major share of the costs of running the services, which were increasing substantially every year; it was therefore desirable to have a new administrative framework to combine national and local interests across an inter-county basis. It was clear that county level was too small an area for hospital services (Curry, 1990). In setting up the health boards, consideration was given to the area, the size of population, and the regions delimited for local government planning and development. The health boards were made up of a majority of elected representatives from local corporations/councils, professionals involved in the provision of health care, and some nominees of the Minister for Health.

The powers of the health boards broke down into mandatory and discretionary powers. Under Section 45 of the Act, health boards were required to make various services available, while in certain other instances, they could exercise discretion to do so. Entitlement to the various services was dependent on whether an individual qualified for full eligibility or limited eligibility. The individuals who qualified for the former, 31 per cent of the population, were holders of a medical card. This group was entitled to all health services free of charge for themselves and their dependants. The remainder of the population, who qualified for limited eligibility, were entitled to a more limited range of services. The health boards were required to provide maternity care for free to all mothers for example. On the other hand, they had discretion to make arrangements for the supply, without charge, of drugs and medicines to persons suffering from a prescribed disability of a long-term or permanent nature (Curry, 1990).

Since the health boards' inception, many carers have been involved in bureaucratic battles in trying to secure Medical Cards for their sons or daughters. Medical cards entitled the user to a full range of services including general practitioner services, prescribed drugs and medicines, in-patient and out-patient public hospital services including consultants' services. Because most community health and social services were not underpinned by any statutory requirements, there was no absolute entitlement, as such, for most services even though a person may have been legally eligible (McMahon and Barron, 2004). Furthermore, for carers there was little official information available on the extent of availability of services across the various health boards or across community care units within the health boards (McMahon and Barron, 2004).

The home-help service was also established under Section 61 of the *Health Act* (1970) and was greatly expanded since its establishment. Access to this service was also at the discretion of health boards, thus its development was constrained by the absence of an adequate legal basis (Curry, 1990). Although the service was mainly provided by the health boards, there was large voluntary sector involvement (O'Louglin, 1999). It consisted predominantly of female workers employed on a part-time basis with low rates of pay and little training.

Even after the *Health Act* (1970) created the community care structures, many voluntary organisations retained a great deal of autonomy in the development and delivery of services. This was due in no small part to a number of older and larger voluntary organisations receiving their funding not by means of 'Section 65 grants' (payments from the earlier *Health Act* (1953)), but directly from the Department of Health. Amongst these organisations were Daughters of Charity Services and Brothers of Charity Services. These organisations became significant providers of services on a national basis and the direct and centralised funding of them arguably allowed them to maintain a powerful and autonomous status.

In relation to community care, the McKinsey Report, *Towards Better Health Care – Management in the Health Board* (1970) recommended that teams be drawn from all those engaged in field services including doctors, nurses, dentists, social workers, health inspectors and assistance officers. They would bring to the family and the individual the concerted efforts of a team rather than the fragmented work of individuals from different services. This system would lead to the devolution of services, the discontinuation of centralised specialist groups and the formation of new multi-disciplinary teams, each to be headed by a director of community care (Curry, 1990).

The Community Care Programme since covers a wide range of services and has three sub-programmes: community protection (health immunisation), community health services (primary care) and community welfare, the latter which includes a range of cash payments (domiciliary care allowance), home help service, and grants to voluntary welfare organisations (Curry, 1990). There was considerable investment in the fields of health at this time. However, this did not challenge Catholic principles because the state limited its role to the provision of resources. As a result, private and voluntary institutions, under the tutelage of the Catholic Church, retained the strategic role of delivering these social goods (McLaughlin, 1993). This meant that services were still imbued with Catholic social principles and little or no statutory regulation.

As the role of state services increased, that of the Parent and Friends Associations did not diminish; it in fact also increased. Generally the pattern was that these voluntary organisations provided the essential services, with the state becoming involved in a supportive role at a later stage. The pioneering role remained relevant as new social problems emerged and as others were redefined. Furthermore, even if it were desirable, it was and still remains highly unlikely that the state could afford to replace the work of voluntary organisations completely. While the voluntary sector had and continues to have obvious strengths, one of the inherent weaknesses of the system was that there was an uneven geographic spread of organisations: while some areas were relatively well served by voluntary groups, others were less so, as later found by the NDA (2004). A further weakness was the lack of financial or general accountability found in many cases (Curry, 1990).

Community Care Implementation Gap (1980–1989)

By the 1980s, Ireland had developed a heavy dependence on multi-national corporations, but as a consequence of changing global economic conditions, they began to withdraw from Ireland. When combined with tensions and contradictions generated by state policies, unemployment levels began to increase dramatically (McLaughlin, 1993). In the face of serious economic difficulties of this time the welfare effort dwindled and disability services were decimated. The deep recession of the 1980s forced the Fine Gael supporters to adopt a more self-interested approach, thus abandoning much of their previous concern for equitable redistribution (McLaughlin, 1993).

Voluntary community action became very vocal and proactive forcing disadvantaged issues onto the wider political agenda. For example, the Alzheimer Society of Ireland was set up in 1982 and was one of the first organisations to officially recognise and target their services towards carers. In terms of social services, the increasing role of the EU began to have a significant influence. For instance, a traditional feature of the Irish income maintenance system was once a claimant has established entitlement, payments were also generally made in respect of any adult and child dependants. Therefore spouses (mostly married women) were regarded as being financially dependent. This was modified following the implementation of an EC Directive in 1986 on the equal treatment of men and women (Curry, 1990).

Much ignorance surrounded disability and these changing times led to a plethora of reports concerning disability services in Ireland; the NESC Report 50, on *Major Issues in Planning Services for Mentally and Physically Handicapped Persons* (1980), *Report of the Working Party on Services for the Mentally Handicapped* (1980), and the Green Paper, *Services for Disabled People towards a Full Life* (1984). Many attempts were made throughout the decade to create a policy document on the scope and structure of welfare services and the respective roles in planning and provision of these services (Curry, 1990). About the same time, the NESC Report No. 84, *Community Care Services: An Overview* (1987) argued that the community care legislation was not specific about entitlement to home-help services, meals-on-wheels, day care facilities for the elderly and other services to name but a few. It was recognised however, that laying down eligibility criteria in legislation could have expenditure implications as it may increase the use of services.

When Fianna Fáil regained government in 1987 it announced that it was essential to reduce the national debt and that there would be public service redundancies, privatisation and public expenditure cutbacks. However, it differed from England in this regard, in that then Taoiseach Charles Haughey made it clear that this retrenchment agenda would be carried out by agreement and national consensus rather than conflict (McLaughlin, 1993). This was carried out by a partnership of the 'social partners' of the state – the Irish Congress of Trade Unions, the employers and the farmers – under the *Programme for National Recovery* launched in October 1987.

Alongside the government's role in providing support for carers, the voluntary sector still continued to be the largest source of services and support for family carers. In addition, two national carer organisations were established in Ireland. Firstly, the Carers Association was set up in 1987 and became the first national carers association for lobbying government. The following year, Caring for Carers Ireland was established by Soroptimist International, a world-wide rights organisation for women, to promote the wellbeing of family carers and those for whom they care.

For carers, the decrease in the numbers in asylum care did not mean that community care was being adequately provided. Rather than being well-coordinated and methodical, Ireland's de-institutionalisation policy and practice was uncoordinated, piecemeal and ad hoc (Amnesty International, 2003). The *Report of the Working Party on Services for the Mentally Handicapped* (1980) highlighted that there were 2,307 people with a learning disability in Ireland in need of accommodation outside of family care (Redmond, 1996: 40). The government approach was that death and the passage of time would eventually reduce the numbers of 'mentally handicapped' in the mental hospitals. Reallocating them to their family home was not possible with the link between those inside the institutions and their families long since gone for many of its members.

The most significant problem with the process of de-institutionalisation was the lack of sufficient resources made available to ease the transition to community care. For example, although the *Social Welfare Act* (1989) paid the Prescribed Relative's Allowance directly to the carer, the payment remained very restrictive and very small financially (£IR27 a week at the time) (Dáil Éireann, 1989). Meanwhile, the reduction of those in asylum care was helped along with better and more specific diagnosis practices which meant that those with intellectual disabilities were filtered out of the same bracket as those with mental health problems. Moreover, *Planning for the Future* 1984 made a provision to move all remaining people with intellectual disabilities to separate 'de-designated' wards within psychiatric hospitals, thereby removing any mandatory requirements for government inspections of these new units. This also meant an abrupt end in data regarding people with intellectual disabilities on where they were displaced.

The National Economic and Social Council (NESC) examined a number of community care services and concluded that wide variations in the level of services for the 'handicapped' could be attributed to the lack of national guidelines on the appropriate level of service, the lack of national uniform criteria of eligibility for certain services, and the discretionary nature of some services (1987). Nor was there a commitment to make the necessary resources available (Curry, 1990). Community care services in Ireland were therefore plagued by lack of investment during this time.

Reform Takes Root (1990–1997)

The reform process began in the 1990s with the 'Celtic Tiger' economic boom mid-decade, a weakening of the ideological power of the Church due to their teachings falling out of touch with a modern Ireland, and the increasing influence of the EU. This period saw the first signs of reform in the areas of health, disability and carer policy. However, while this period saw the introduction of some state-run services and the taking over of some services run by voluntary and charity groups, the welfare drive did not resume with the relative prosperity of the time, as the new wealth was not channelled into an additional welfare effort. Investment in welfare and health care was largely catch-up funding in infrastructure and services.

Along with its fellow EU member states, there were also social changes such as the increasing proportion of married women in the workforce, which had implications for the provision of family care for those with intellectual disabilities. This raised new issues for a policy of community-based care which was built on the assumption of availability and willingness on the part of one section of society to forego gainful employment in order to provide largely unsupported care. According to Quin et al. (2005: 2) this assumed altruism was a good example of how social policies could be based on expectations and assumptions about what is appropriate and desirable.

The *Social Welfare Act* (1990), under TD Michael Woods, introduced a means-tested 'Carer's Allowance' (CA). The CA has since been a social assistance payment payable to someone who resides with or has a direct link with, and provides full-time care to a person who is so incapacitated as to require full-time care. The payment is very much constructed as an earnings substitution, prohibiting the carer from engaging in employment (also assets). In the case of married carers, disregard of spouse's income was introduced in 1994 (£IR100) and gradually increased. Those in receipt of the Carers allowance also get a free companion travel pass, free telephone rental, TV licence, and gas/electricity. However, unlike in the UK, this is a means tested payment making eligibility very difficult.

That same year, the report *Needs and Abilities* (Department of Health, 1990) outlined the main service developments to enable people with an intellectual disability to live in their local communities with support services to meet their needs. For the first time, there was a strong acknowledgement of family care, noting that 'many families happily continue to care for their son or daughter well into their adult years' (p. 37). The emphasis was on helping families to resolve or alleviate the difficulties which may inhibit them from caring. However, the report completely underestimated the numbers still living in large congregated settings, thus failing to kick-start a development in community focused care:

> We have been fortunate in Ireland that our residential centres have generally been small by international standards and many have never had the institutional characteristics which have been a feature of such centres in a number of developed countries.[7]

The recommendations were met with a shiftless and ineffective response by service providers. Without the short-term injection of funding, the aims of the report largely faltered.

Health Board Coordinating Committees were established for services for people with intellectual disability which included representatives of the health boards, voluntary agencies and clients/parents. It since became a requirement for the Department of Health and Children to work in a partnership with providers of health care, and other departments and bodies. This gave carer organisations and carers themselves a voice. At the time, the Carers' Charter was launched in 1991 by Caring for Carers Ireland, outlining a call for the rights underpinning the needs of carers. Since the charter was launched, most progress in addressing carers' issues has been based on its recommendations. However, a Carers' Strategy never became enshrined by government, which meant the charter has remained an aspirational document.

In terms of disability legislation, Ireland was a late starter. In November 1993 the Minister for Equality and Law Reform, Mervyn Taylor, TD, established a *Commission on the Status of People with Disabilities*. The terms of reference underpinning the appointment of the commission included: 'to advise the Government on practical measures necessary to ensure that people with a disability

---

7 Review Group on Mental Handicap Services 1990 *Needs and Abilities: A Policy for the Intellectually Disabled*. Stationery Office, Dublin. p. 39.

can exercise their rights to participate, to the fullest extent of their potential, in economic, social and cultural life; to examine the organisation and adequacy of existing services, both public and voluntary, to meet their needs; and to establish the estimated costs of all recommendations made' (Commission on the Status of People with Disabilities, 1996).

While the Commission was deliberating, the 1994 *Health Strategy* led to the establishment of the National Intellectual Disability Database, which was introduced in order to identify unmet needs, provide a service planning tool and a mechanism for monitoring progress. In addition, various services were developed for specific groups of people with intellectual disability. Because of the voluntary nature of the database the information contained within it has since not been as comprehensive as hoped; but it began to close the information gap required for service planning.

In terms of the voluntary sector, Care Alliance Ireland was set up in 1995 as an umbrella organisation to provide a means for voluntary organisations concerned with the needs of carers to work together for the development and promotion of policies and strategies to meet such needs. According to a spokesperson for the organisation (Respondents have been abbreviated to R.):

> Care Alliance Ireland came about simply because [Paul] at the time was CEO of the Health Board and he said if you're hoping to progress, to get services and support and funding for Carers, instead of having all of these different itsy-bitsy groups that if we could come together and speak with one voice, because it is for carers, to benefit carers, that we would be in a much stronger position. (R. Caring for Carers Ireland)

Therefore Care Alliance Ireland became a network and facilitator for the other regional carer groups. More centrally, their task has been to lobby in order to keep the issues in front of government. Also, by the mid-1990s, the other carer voluntary groups – Caring for Carers and the Carer's Association – had developed an extensive national spread of regional centres delivering local services such as home-help and information, as well as their advocacy role.

During the same period, some concern had arisen from the *Enhancing the Partnership* Report (1997) regarding the direct funding of some voluntary agencies by the Department of Health and Children, arguing that it impeded the proper co-ordination and development of services at a local level. Hence, it was agreed that funding for *all* voluntary bodies would be provided through the health boards on the basis of service agreements (1998 when fully implemented). The Report's working group also noted that Section 26, though not widely used, offered a better framework than Section 65 to support the kind of relationship to be expressed in service agreements between the health boards and voluntary groups. Section 26 of the *Health Act* (1970) enabled the health boards to enter into arrangements with voluntary organisations to provide services on their behalf. By specifying the conditions in the regulations, they were given a statutory basis

(Disability Federation of Ireland, 2002). However, despite this recommendation, most voluntary organisations preferred the looser controlled Section 65 funding.

On 18 November 1996, the *Report of The Commission on the Status of People with Disabilities – A Strategy for Equality* was published. Significantly they found that people with disabilities, including persons with intellectual disabilities, were the neglected citizens of Ireland. Many submissions mentioned the lack of co-ordination between service providers, the fragmentation of services and the difficulty in getting entitlements. Deficits in education, employment and training, income support, health and personal support and the ongoing strains, physical, emotional and social, which long-term carers experience were also brought to the fore (Commission on the Status of People with Disabilities, 1996). Some recommendations more directly supported family carers, such as the expansion of the home help scheme and respite care services and national standards for services for people with disabilities in the community. The report was highly critical of many of the social barriers, negative attitudes and poor quality of outmoded services, which created marginalisation. The absence of services in the health and social care field were highlighted in the report; '...people with disabilities, parents and carers have serious concerns as to the quality of some existing services, and about the lack of some fundamental services' (1996:161).

The Commission believed it necessary to create an executive body which would monitor the impact of public policy and services on people with disability and argued they should have the power to intervene in particular cases in order to ensure equity. It was against this backdrop that the Commission recommended the establishment of a National Disability Authority which would report to the Department of Equality and Law Reform (now the Department of Justice, and Law Reform). This Report brought a new chapter to disability and carer policy in Ireland and arguably brought the issue of rights to the mainstream.

Modernisation and Civil Renewal (1997–1999)

Fianna Fáil returned to power in 1997 under the leadership of Bertie Ahern, in coalition with the Progressive Democrats and, with one subsequent change in Taoiseach, have been in power since. In 1997, Brian Cowen was appointed Minister for Health and Children. Addressing identified needs in intellectual disability services was one of his top priorities. The Department of Health document, *Services to Persons with a Mental Handicap/Intellectual Disability: An Assessment of Need 1997–2001*, showed that there was a requirement for 1,036 extra places in day services and 1,439 extra places in respite/residential care in Ireland (DoHC, 1997). He approved funding of £IR240,000 to the Independent Living Community Services to help it defray accumulated debts. He also approved a grant of £IR130,000 to the Centre for Independent Living. The Minister for Social, Community and Family Affairs, Dermot Ahern, also approved a package of funding of £IR4,325,000 which directly benefited people with physical and sensory disabilities and voluntary agencies (Dáil Éireann, 1997). The extra funding for respite places were welcomed by family carers who had been struggling with limited supports from under funded voluntary organisations. The Parent and Friends Associations also began to receive more government support.

The Fianna Fáil government, largely led by the EU, also advocated a renewed emphasis on the role of the voluntary sector. It published a Green Paper, *Supporting Voluntary Activity* in May 1997, as part of the National Anti-Poverty Strategy (Government of Ireland, 1997). It promoted openness, accountability and transparency and also proposed principles to apply to the funding of the voluntary and community sector. It elevated this area of social activity to a new level of importance in public discourse. At the time it was reckoned by the Green Paper that 'the voluntary sector had the potential to create a vibrant civil and active society' (Powell and Guerin, 1997). This led to Partnership 2000, which consisted of 38 area-based partnership companies funded by the EU and the national government. These were envisaged as locally-based companies consisting of 'community interests, state development agency executives, Health Board and local authority officials and social partner representatives' (Programme for Economic and Social Progress, 1991: 77). The aim was to combine statutory, voluntary and other social partners in an effort to combat social and economic exclusion. According to Powell (1998: 25):

> civil society connected to generative political strategies, based on more complex ideas of equality and a more empowering concept of citizenship, is a vibrant and powerful concept of civic renewal in an era of social fragmentation.

With the National Anti-Poverty Strategy (1997–2007), Partnership 2000 (1997–2000) and the courting of the community sector by elected politicians, this involvement began to take a more central role. Clearly, as with any sector, a jockeying of power within organisations and between organisations took place. The voluntary groups also had to be aware of repercussions on the client base where struggles could ensue to see who was going to represent their interests, and whether it was done effectively or not (Donoghue, 1998). Organisations representing women, youth, travellers, disability, unemployment, the environment and rural development were all included in Partnership 2000. Carers however were left out of the partnership process which raised serious issues about their lobbying potential. Whatever their role as support providers, it seemed pertinent that they would have a voice at the partnership level. However, more generally, according to Donoghue (1998), many in the voluntary sector felt that participation did not lead to policy but only to procedures. In addition, Comhairle was set up to promote and support voluntary organisations. It set up the Resource Database for the Voluntary and Community Sector in Ireland (Comhairle, 2001).

In 1999, the *Health (Eastern Regional Health Authority) Act* finally established three Area Health Boards and an Eastern Regional Health Authority which would oversee the operation of those Boards (Disability Federation of Ireland, 2002). Under the terms of the *Health (ERHA) Act* (1999) the Health Board Executive

(HeBE) was specifically established to further improve the efficiency and effectiveness of health and personal social services. HeBE began to undertake conjointly, activities falling within the executive remit of the health boards, area health boards and the ERHA. The HeBE reflected the Executive's commitment to a modernisation agenda for the State's health delivery system. Their functions included a spectrum of operational activities which were previously undertaken by the Department of Health and Children. Rather than another management layer above the health boards, it saw itself as a complementary body which enabled the various health boards work together to progress a national health agenda.

In November 1999, Brian Cowen, allocated £IR594m in gross expenditure to disability services. The objective for disability services was to significantly reduce the waiting lists, in addition to having enhanced the level of respite care available, over the next two years. As a result of the investment made in these services over 900 residential/respite places and over 900 day places were put in place (Department of Health and Children, 2000). For at least the last twenty years, every Minister for Finance had made an allocation in the Budget to enable new places to be created, and some in-roads had been made in the waiting lists. As a result of Brian Cowen's aim to put existing disability services on a more secure financial footing, the amount allocated was quite substantial, and there was a great deal of hope in the community that continuation of that plan would begin to see the numbers on waiting lists decline. However, as the following section shows, because of the 'relaxed-control' model which Ireland had developed with an historical reluctance to manage the disability and carer service landscape hands-on, reform remained frustratingly hindered.

Structural Change (2000–Present)

The period from 2000 to the present has been characterised by much structural change in the community care landscape. However, although carers' identities by this time had become increasingly more visible, the State's role in providing support has remained unclear. In recognition of the large voluntary sector, the State's attention has been spent on redefining the sector and their relationship with it. According to one Independent Teachta Dáila.[8]

> We have to get away from the idea of charity. The charity-based idea was rampant in Irish Society. It's a historical thing, it's a cultural thing. So we've got to move towards a rights based approach and respect people and also the whole idea of accommodating difference (Independent TD).

8 Irish Government Minister of Parliament.

The Green Paper *Supporting Voluntary Activity* finally became a White Paper *A Framework for Supporting Voluntary Activity*[9] (DoHC, 2000). Despite its recommendations for jointly developed service agreements, these still read like high-level, somewhat abstract guidelines that merely describe the ideal principles of engagement, in broad terms. In practice, these do not specify details of how to structure relationships. Monitoring is thus rare and, where it is in place, is poorly carried out. As Donoghue (2007) notes, the White Paper exists more in the realm of rhetoric than practice in today's service provision. A significant change in support for the voluntary sector was announced in the 2001 Budget. This involved giving tax relief to voluntary and community organisations who met certain conditions (and to a number of other bodies as well). This general scheme incorporated most of the pre-existing schemes but applied much more widely.

In January 2000, a party re-shuffle appointed Brian Cowen as Minister for Foreign Affairs and Michéal Martin as new Minister for Health and Children. While 900 residential and 400 respite places had been provided, a further 3,000 people were still awaiting a service. The 2000 Budget introduced a significant injection of new funding for intellectual disability services and in health more generally (O'Connell, 2000). In November 2001, the Department of Health and Children launched *The Health Strategy, Quality and Fairness – A Health System For You*. This contained proposals for significant reform of the health service towards a more integrated and person-centred approach, emphasising the provision of services in a non-discriminatory and inclusive way (Department of Health and Children, 2001). For people with intellectual disabilities in particular, it outlined the expansion of residential care places, more day, community, respite care and support services; to complete the programme to transfer people with an intellectual disability currently in psychiatric hospitals to appropriate (group home) accommodation no later than the end of 2006, and investment in support services for people with autism, including an information database on the numbers of persons with autism and their service needs. Key points for the care of people with intellectual disabilities included: 7,000 day centre places to be provided; Recruitment of staff to improve 600 additional day hospital beds with specialist treatment; 800 additional extended care places per annum over the next seven years including provision for people with dementia; and improved staffing levels in extended care units. The report went further in identifying new investment to increase capacity through an expansion of community based services. By the end of 2002 the following commitments had been made under Quality and Fairness (DoHC, 2001): €38m for existing services and identified needs; €25m for the development of new services (100 new residential places, 75 new respite places, 600 new day places, support services, transfer from inappropriate placements); and €1.27m under the National Development Plan for ongoing capital projects (McMahon and Barron, 2004).

9 'A Framework for Supporting Voluntary Activity and for Developing the Relationship between the State and the Community and the Voluntary Sector'.

Since the earlier 1996 Commission on the Status of Persons with Disabilities, disability rights had entered into the lexicon of people with disabilities and their organisations. Many national organisations began pushing for a wider statutory basis for the protection of human rights of people with disabilities in Ireland, with an emphasis on the delivery of services and equality as a right. This led to a new raft of disability legislative measures. The Equality Authority was set up as an independent body under the *Employment Equality Act* (1998) to prohibit discrimination in relation to employment, training and related areas on nine grounds, one of which was disability. Their role was to promote and defend the rights established in this equality legislation. They were instrumental for getting *The Equal Status Act* (2000) enshrined which prohibited discrimination in relation to the supply of goods, facilities and services, thus giving families of young adults with intellectual disabilities much needed non-discrimination protection in their arsenal.

A *Disability Bill* was also drafted in 2001. However, it offered no social rights to those in need of the services to actually seek redress if the services are not provided. It therefore became a contentious issue among disability groups and was one of the most hotly debated pieces of legislation for a long time in the Oireachtas.[10] With much outrage from the disability organisations, it was withdrawn in order to be re-drafted. The government fear was that the costs associated with implementing it were prohibitive.

While the Bill was being re-considered, the *Carer's Leave Act* (2001) was introduced to make it possible for workers to take a temporary choice of becoming a carer without loss of employment. It therefore has gone some way towards recognising the need for flexibility in employment. However, even though many people availing of Carer's Leave provisions would be entitled to Carer's Benefit, it is likely to be used only by those in secure employment. The Act therefore, fails to address the situation of those who are in the most unfavourable position financially, e.g., those in temporary work or without sufficient Pay Related Social Insurance (PRSI) contributions (Comhairle, July 2002).

This reluctance to adequately support carers can be perhaps explained by the tax policy of Fianna Fáil and the Progressive Democrats. Both parties made it clear that they did not want the high tax rates of the Labour party in the 1980s. They have since been committed to a low taxation, low government spending economy, unlike the social democratic countries in Europe like France and Germany. As a result, the Irish middle classes have begun more recently to move away from the public health system towards private health insurance because the public system is not delivering the quality of services expected. According to Sweeney (2004), the government has consciously decided not to fund the public health care system because it does not want to raise the taxes which are needed to pay for modern health. For example, in the launch of the Book of Estimates November 2002, the Minister for Finance stated that attention should be focused on 'the value we are

10 Irish Parliament.

getting in terms of the quality and quantity of public services' rather than on the creation of new services (National Disability Authority, 2004: 53).

However, although the Government has the lowest taxes in Europe, it is wrong to state that Ireland is a low-tax economy. While it has the lowest taxes as a percentage of GDP, Ireland is not a low-tax economy for most of its citizens; it is a medium-tax country for most and it is an extraordinarily low-tax country for some (Sweeney, 2004). It is the imbalance in the way tax is raised which is the problem. Firstly, Ireland has high taxes on spending, in the form of VAT, and on low incomes. Secondly, there are a myriad of exemptions and loopholes in the tax system which allow legal avoidance for those on higher incomes, such as property investment for nursing homes for example. The government gives a total tax write-off to investors in property. The tax forgone from avoidance amounts to hundreds of millions and could pay for the capital and current needs of non-congregated community care. As the flight of the middle classes from public health services grows, the services get worse, and the Government cuts spending more (Sweeney, 2004).

In 2003 there was no allocation made for new services and places in disability support. Despite an expansion in funding since 1997, the 2003 budget provided only for the maintenance of existing levels of service. This was despite 2003 being the European Year of People with Disabilities. This led to a lengthy public campaign by individual organisations throughout the country, national representative umbrella groups like NAMHI, the Federation of Voluntary Bodies, the Forum of People with Disabilities and others. This campaign resulted in the Government coming up with a package of €20m for people with disabilities in July 2003 (NAMHI, August 2003). The new funding consisted of €15m for services to persons with intellectual disability and autism for emergency residential placement, the provision of day services for young adults who had left school and the enhancement of health related support services for children. Another €45m was allocated to services for persons with physical or sensory disabilities.

Later that year, there was an additional €25m provided to support persons with intellectual, physical or sensory disabilities, announced by Minister McCreevy on December 2003. However, a discourse of 'unmet residential need' had come to prominence from the disability support sector. This was largely driven by a new emphasis on person-centred planning which focused on individual service placements, rather than on natural supported living arrangements. This arguably led to a disconnect between many individuals with disabilities and their own families. Service providers were intent on offering more group home placements. Meanwhile, with limited family support options available and a paternalistic, overly clinical disability sector, families were being led to believe that a wrap-around 'cradle to grave' service was more desirable. As a result, the extra funding was used to provide for more residential placements.

By this time, the traditional discourses regarding disability being a charity issue had decidedly changed. All these increases made some inroads into waiting lists, however the government found that the Budget did not have the expected impact on the waiting list for day or residential services of over 2,300 people with intellectual disabilities (NAMHI newsletter, 2004). While greater sums may well have been invested in these times, it was largely making up for the cutbacks in the 1980s. The government was also faced with the prospect of people with disabilities living longer than ever before. However, there was a deeper infrastructural issue at the root of this problem, which was halting much progress in the modernisation of Ireland's landscape of care. This would be discovered the following year in a national audit of the sector.

In the mean time, on 18 June 2003, the Government announced a major reform programme for the Irish health services. Given that disability services are provided through the health service, this was considered to be the most extensive reform programme in over 30 years. The focus of the reform was largely improved health care management. This was considered to be necessary to create modern and responsive health services that were able to deliver on the health strategy and the increasingly complex demands placed on the health care system. This was particularly important for disability services, which were often fragmented and poorly planned due to a range of management, organisational and resource problems (National Disability Authority, 2004).

The change was led by a plethora of major reports on the Irish health structures, including amongst others, the Prospectus Report (2003) and the Hanly Report (2003). The Prospectus Report carried out an audit of structures and functions in the health system on behalf of the Department of Health and Children. The Hanly Report was carried out by the National Task Force on Medical Staffing to improve primary patient care. The two reports showed that the current system was ineffective, cumbersome and fragmented. They recommended, first, that rationalisation, standardisation and improved co-ordination were needed to overcome fragmentation. Second, that more clarity was needed about roles and decision-making. Third, effective planning processes should ensure that people were at the centre of care by linking needs assessment, planning of services, funding and activity. They advocated a major rationalisation of existing health service agencies, including the abolition of the existing Health Board structures and the consolidation and amalgamation of the existing 32 agencies (made up of health boards, the Eastern Regional Health Authority and hospital providers) and the establishment of a Health Service Executive to manage and deliver the health service as a single national service (National Disability Authority, 2004).

With Mary Harney as Minister for Health and Children (2004–), the reform programme, following the reports, introduced major changes in the structure and organisation of health services. These documents all gave attention to issues relevant for carers, including more support for community services to help dependant people remain in their own homes. Support for carers was also typically alluded to, and consultations subsequently began between government and carer organisations to develop a Carers Strategy. There was a lack of a statutory basis for many of the services that had central relevance for carers, and also an absence of clear links between eligibility and entitlement to these services. This left considerable scope for anomaly and inequity in access to services. The fact that the service delivery model was a residual one, with the 'availability' of a carer or carers taken into consideration in rationing scarce services, coupled with the fact that carers were seldom direct clients of the health and social services, added to the potential for anomaly and inequity (McMahon and Barron, 2004). The result of the reports brought a new era in the health service, with the *Health Act* (2004). From 1 January 2005, the day to day running of services was handed over by the Department of Health and health boards to a new body called the Health Service Executive (HSE) and the Health Service Executive Areas (HSEAs) (Donnellan, 2004). The HSE has four regional offices and a headquarters in Naas, however the Health Service Executive Areas retained directors of finance and other services from the health boards in an extensive interim period (Donnellan, 2004). The *Health Act* also brought the developmental and coordinating committees to a close.

In terms of the funding contracts within the new HSE structure, there were two new funding streams of block grants available through the HSE which disability agencies were able to apply for. These were established through separate sections of the 2004 Health Act:

- Section 38 grants (old Section 26 funded organisations) related to agencies/groups providing services on behalf of the HSE. This referred to services which the HSE was legally and statutorily required to provide and enter into an arrangement with an outside agency to do so on its behalf.
- Section 39 funding (old Section 65 funded organisations) related to agencies/groups undertaking services which were similar or ancillary to those of the HSE and to whom the HSE was providing grant aid to do so. However the HSE would not be legally or statutorily obligated to provide such services.

In terms of Section 38 funding, there has been an expectation that those in receipt of the grant are quasi-governmental (generally non-profit) organisations, who deliver essential supports on behalf of the HSE. This has meant that the staffing, levels of pay, management etc are more directly influenced by government, for example state embargo's on new employment positions. This is limited to 26 agencies currently within the HSE Employment Control Framework. However, there is a range of activities carried out within organisations that could fall under either definition as outlined above (Section 38 and 39) (Disability Federation of Ireland, 2009). For instance, many organisations that developed out of Parents and Friends Associations, but provide equally essential services, are often under the Section 39 funding stream, whereas many larger non-statutory 'Church based' organisations fit under Section 38.

The year following the *Health Act*, the government finally enacted the *Disability Act* (2005). This led to a process of mainstreaming of disability issues across government departments and sectoral plans (disability progress plans for 6 government departments). This was the cornerstone of the government's National Disability Strategy which also saw the implementation of a multi-annual funding programme for the disability support sector over a period of three years. While this had some success, in terms of more residential 'group home' placements in the sector, much of the multi-annual funding was wasted because of other priorities and deficits within the newly formed HSEAs (Disability Federation of Ireland, 2008). The Disability Act led to much disappointment within the Irish disability movement. Many disability organisations felt let down by the lack of statutory rights in the legislation, particularly after the level of consultation with the government during the drafting stage. People with disabilities and their families were forced to re-think their focus on a discourse of rights as a tool for lobbying government. In the end, government was happy to promote 'rights' (non-discrimination, equality etc.) but was fearful and reluctant to enshrine 'a right' to a service.

While this drama was unfolding, a ground-breaking audit by the Comptroller and Auditor General (C&AG) of the disability service landscape was published which finally exposed the effects of the government's reluctance to regulate or monitor the disability support sector (2005). As identified earlier, despite the money spent on disability services throughout the 1990s and early 2000s, there was a deeper infrastructural issue halting progress in modernising disability services. The audit revealed evidence of the lenient relationship between government and voluntary service providers. Its report found a widespread failure among voluntary bodies, many of which were secular, to provide audited financial statements or disclose levels of executive pay. The audit of 42 non-profit organisations between November 2004 and January 2005 found that 12 groups did not file accounts for 2003. In particular, one large organisation which received €288m during 2000–2004 had not provided financial statements for these four years. It identified that the State's relationship with nonprofit organisations had evolved into one where services to persons with disabilities were the result of an historical pattern of provision and were largely negotiated rather than the result of contested procurement. As was seen with the White Paper, *Supporting Voluntary Activity* (2000), the current approach to the funding of nonprofit organisations is based on high-level framework documents with global funding and incremental increases. The risk with this approach is that the core funding allocation may over time become weakly linked to levels of identified need and as a result, funding may not always be targeted to areas of greatest need. In contrast to the trend in the US and UK towards more formal, market-style purchaser-provider contracts for managing the relationship between state and nonprofit organisations (see Milligan and Conradson, 2006), Ireland's model has continued its long history of operating a relatively decentralised and ad-hoc approach to managing such providers, particularly in the disability sector.

In 2006, the government made an ambitious agenda for social change, with a ten-year social partnership agreement 'Towards 2016'. This develops a new framework to address key social challenges, which the individual faces at each stage of life. This means a focus on the needs of children, young adults, people of working age, older people and people with disabilities. This approach proposes that public services will need to be designed around individuals and their requirements, rather than based on different administrative boundaries.

This approach will take time to deliver and the agreement sets out how Ireland should measure and review progress over a ten-year framework agreement (Government of Ireland, 2006).

As part of 'Towards 2016' and under the Programme for Government in 2007, a National Carers Strategy was promised by the Government. It set up a consultation in the development of a National Carers' Strategy. It encouraged members of the public to participate in submissions for the strategy, which would 'set out the Government's vision for family and informal carers and establish a set of goals and actions in areas such as income support, health care and services' (Department of Social Protection, 2009). However, in 2009 with the recent economic recession, the government withdrew from the National Carers' Strategy. The Department of Social and Family Affairs released a statement stating (2009) that it would not be publishing the strategy because of the economic situation. Minister Mary Hanafin said any submissions that were made during the consultation process would be considered in any future plans. However, in the statement, she said the economic situation 'makes it difficult to commit to major advances in services for carers.' Ms Hanafin said she appreciated the decision not to publish the strategy would be disappointing for carers and the people for whom they care. In response, Fine Gael Social and Family Affairs Spokeswoman Olwyn Enright accused Ms Hanafin of trying to bury her decision to axe the National Carers' Strategy by timing the announcement with the release of poor Exchequer figures:

> This is an appalling decision from Minister Hanafin and is an act of betrayal after years of promises. But just as bad is her decision to time the announcement with the release of some of the worst Exchequer figures ever seen in Ireland. This is a clear attempt by the Minister to bury the news. The Government has known for weeks that the new Exchequer figures were likely to be very devastating. More than 161,000 carers across Ireland had pinned their hopes on the promise to set up a National Carers' Strategy, as set out in the Programme for Government, and supposed to be up and running by the end of 2007. The Government failed to meet this target in 2007 and is now hiding behind the current economic situation (quoted in *The Irish Times*, 3 March 2009).

While the economic situation is certainly a major constraint to a renewed policy agenda, it begs the question why the government failed to implement any carers' strategy during the previous ten years, during the economic boom, dubbed by many as the 'Celtic Tiger'.

Similarly, the disability sector is currently in a difficult climate. Disability services currently exist at a crossroads in the wake of the earlier audit and subsequent partnership strategy. The government have since begun a major review to identify inefficiences in the sector on one hand, and modernise community support in line with international best-practice on the other. The transformation challenges are significant given the long-standing legacies and re-organisation fatigue within the sector. Yet the government have been determined to modernise the sector 'within' the same budget, and the HSE have commissioned a day service review and a congregated settings review. However, despite the earlier audit, the government remain reluctant to introduce mandatory standards for regulating the sector, for fears that it will be too costly for the state.

Conclusion

From analysing the Irish welfare state, it is clear that Ireland has developed very differently to England and in particular the US. Above all, the social construction of the traditional family unit as the cornerstone of society was even more pronounced in Ireland. Thus the key characteristics of the Irish care support model is the pivotal role of family caregivers, and the very restricted role of state in the provision of care services for either the carer or the care recipient, with welfare dominated by charities and voluntary sector involvement. In contrast to the other two comparative jurisdictions, Ireland has developed neither the extended social rights accorded to people with disabilities in the US nor the widespread landscape of social services in England, preferring a 'relaxed-control' model of commissioning services (Power and Kenny, in press). At the heart of the Irish system is a narrow, gendered, interpretation of the responsibilities of citizenship. As a result of Ireland's distinct socio-cultural context of care, it serves as a particularly interesting case study in examining broader debates in welfare and redistributive justice for family caregiving.

The chapter followed a similar structure to the two international case-studies, by focusing on legislation and policy, and addressed the changing discourses surrounding disability and family care throughout these times. Carers have been typified in Irish policy by overtly paternalistic assumptions regarding the role of women in the home. Alongside these developments, the institutions still remained a dominant feature of the care landscape, largely juxtaposing the subsidiarity principle of resisting state intervention in family life. When examined more closely however, the infrastructure of state residential care can be seen as a relic of an unwanted Victorian system of care, which the government sought to keep at arm's length from their control. Family care was thus doubly disadvantaged; with a state reluctant to intervene in supporting community life, and a Church reluctant to embrace less congregated forms of care.

More recently, it was possible to see how the state gradually became more involved in family policy as the social construction of disability and care as a charity issue waned. Despite the increases in state expenditures in the sector, the disability sector has remained relatively autonomous and decentralised. As a result, providers have largely set the agenda. With the unique blend of Catholic conservative 'family' policy and 'neo-liberal' statutory provision, the provision of disability and care support in Ireland could be characterised by a 'relaxed-control' approach (Power and Kenny, in press). The main characteristics of this approach are the decentralised regulation of the nonprofit sector, little or no monitoring, and relatively autonomous agencies. Historically, the lack of monitoring benefited the State in that they could depend on the church to carry on with the business of disability provision, without taking upon itself burdens related to the 'problem of the handicapped' (Department of Health, 1960).

Some have noted that these features of voluntary sector governance allow for the inherent potential of voluntary organisations to be more innovative and flexible than larger, state-wide bureaucracies (see Popay et al., 1999; Van Til, 2007). To some extent this may be true in this case, as there is great diversity within the voluntary sector in relation to aims, resources, scope of activity and type of personnel. Some employ full-time paid staff and are entirely funded by statutory grants,[11] others rely on unpaid volunteers, and some have a combination of full-time staff and volunteers. The majority receive some statutory grants, but some still rely on voluntary contributions. There are approximately 214 different organisations, ranging from large-scale service providers, special schools and local volunteer groups. These include mutual support and self-help organisations, local development associations, resource and service-providing organisations, representative and co-ordinating organisations, and campaigning bodies.

Within this medley of associations and groups however, is a lack of shared knowledge between service providers, and from a geographic point of view, it appears that service provision is often planned in a way that only one provider operates per coverage area. Generally, the organisations themselves focus on their local services. Representation has therefore been along geographical or interest lines and only rarely both. Accountability is also an issue as the people who provide the services have been free to do so any way their organisation's philosophy sees fit. Moreover, individuals cannot easily move to another jurisdiction, without having to undergo a new assessment. Clearly there is a whole range of geographical issues such as uneven spatial coverage and unequal access which arise as a result of these restrictions. This has led to a landscape of care in Ireland where there is unequal, or variable, distribution of services geographically with some areas maintaining very traditional support arrangements. This has led many families to have a long-held focus on residential services where those who receive a place are believed to be the 'lucky ones', rather than organisations working with families in developing and sustaining natural supports and a life in the community.

Despite the level of funding recently given to the sector, the overall level of service provision is low among the great majority of carers. Even though some of the services which would meet the needs of carers are in existence, they are not always reaching the carer, and so are not being used effectively to maintain the informal caring relationships. As early as 1987, the National Economic and Social Council in their report, Community Care Services (1987), argued that community care should provide 'a framework of services to families, communities and voluntary organisations to allow them to provide various forms of care'. Unfortunately this

11 Some are 100 per cent funded through Section 38 grants, meaning they are quasi-governmental organisations.

is not the case today as the system is characterised by no national strategy, and a residual belief in the value of a wrap-around 'cradle-to-grave' service from a provider. The next section delves deeper into the Irish landscape of care, to see how family carers themselves are shaped by such a care structure.

PART III
Life Within the Landscape

Chapter 7
Regional Allocation of Irish Care Policy

The previous chapter on carers' policy in Ireland started with a general comparison with England and the US, and went on to analyse how the Irish care system developed in contrast over time. This final part of the book provides a deeper analysis of how the discourses and policy have shaped structures on the ground, with specific reference to the regional allocation of services for carers in Ireland. In this chapter, as well as focusing on the institutional ideologies and frameworks that structure home-care support services, an important component of the analysis is to investigate the experiences of the carers themselves and how the care supports are offered. Evidence is provided through interviews carried out with carer associations as well as carers themselves.[1] Firstly, the analysis focuses on the local infrastructure of care services and the relative roles the statutory health services and non-profit sector play in delivering services. Secondly, it focuses on the narratives of carers regarding their daily experiences of accessing the various forms of support available.

In terms of a contextual background, as explored in the last chapter, the voluntary sector now constitutes a crucial player in the welfare field. Despite this, the central position of the State is still ensured by the fact that it finances most social policy programs. In Ireland at the local level, local authorities bear little or no responsibility for most social security programs. While local authorities participate in the running of some health services, they depend heavily on central grants allocated for specified purposes. More crucially, the Health Service Executive Areas (formerly health boards) are central to the administrative control over community care and service delivery at the regional level. This means that carers are faced with a diverse array of services across different sectors. The following sections thus examine the particular roles each of the sectors play in the landscape of care and the different issues involved.

Facing the Transition: Moving From Education into Adult Services

The transition period at 18 years of age is a traumatic experience for many parents of persons with an intellectual disability as they can no longer rely on special or mainstream education at this stage to provide services or indirectly to gain respite for themselves. The move from adolescence to adulthood for a person with an intellectual disability is particularly difficult, as they and their families have to face

1 Carers are denoted as 'C' in the interview quotes and carer organisations as 'CO'.

the significant concerns over further educational opportunities, job prospects and changes in services. While many families may experience some of these concerns in earlier years, these issues become centrally framed during this transition period. As Redmond (1996) notes, many families with otherwise excellent coping faculties appear to find the period of school leaving far more difficult and stressful than might have been anticipated. Particularly striking is the overall ignorance on the part of many parents about post-school service provision.

At the point of transition, the quality and scope of the child's education becomes a major cause of concern for carers, as many of the opportunities in adult life rely on achieving educational requirements at an earlier age. In addition, families face a transition into a more de-centralised and fragmented spectrum of supports as noted in the *Report of the Review Group on Mental Handicap Services* (1990), which acknowledged that school provides a guaranteed daily break for carers. According to Redmond (1996), for many families, the period from school entry until mid-teens is often a relatively tranquil time where parents may experience an emotional moratorium from the traumas and uncertainties encountered in their child's early years (p. 29).

Many of the carers interviewed had been of the first generation to integrate their sons and daughters into mainstream education. In general, they spoke about the lack of knowledge from those working in schools, and negative attitudes towards those with disabilities right up to and past the transition at 18 years of age:

> [John] did go to mainstream school. He got no help. It was the very beginning of integration back in 1985 and a lot of pressure was put on *not* sending him. So there was no help at any place along the way. You're looked on as not facing the fact that your child has DS [Down's Syndrome] even if you're just *enquiring* if he could go to mainstream. Really, the diagnosis of DS doesn't predict development. But if you're constantly told he'll never do this, then it really does colour your judgement. (C16)

This time in many of the carers' lives had been physically and mentally exhausting because of the problems experienced in trying to gain access to speech and language therapy. The effects of not having access to early intervention was apparent from many parent's observations regarding the development of their adult son or daughter. More fundamentally, many of the carers' concerns were still recent, drawing attention to the current problems facing carers of children with an intellectual disability today. A particular issue, according to the National Disability Authority, has been the shortage of speech and language therapists (2004). This was evident in the study, with many carers speaking of the consequences for their sons or daughters, from not being able to access basic speech and language therapy at an earlier age:

> One disadvantage is that his speech is very bad. There again [he had] no training whatsoever, and I'm sure with speech therapy he could have certainly been

> better…He's always trying to write but he can't write... it looks like a Russian script. (C7)

The long term implications of this for a person moving into adulthood are clear. Without early intervention, many of the independent living aspirations that a person and their family share fail to be realised as the person grows older.

Carers Payments

The issue of payments for carers represents the realm of social rights where much uncertainty has arisen in discourses regarding the role of the state. As discussed, Marshall's (1977) notion of social rights responds to the social inequalities that threaten civil and political citizenship. However, unlike political and civil rights, which have aided the development of capitalism and its class system, social rights are, according to Marshall, seen as being in conflict with capitalism. Unlike contributory insurance therefore, a statutory assistance payment is depicted as involving high levels of state expenditure and intervention, thus in contrast to civil or political rights. Furthermore, as Chapter 3 details, there was a very deliberate separation of male/female, public/private in social rights (O'Brien and Penna, 1998). Caregiving in liberal thought is constructed as very much a private and female enterprise, thus paying carers has always been a contentious issue with neo-liberal government.

In terms of social benefits for carers, the *Carer's Allowance* is regarded as the main payment from the government to acknowledge a carer's work. While many carers had been previously eligible for the *Domiciliary Care Allowance* – a non-means-tested benefit – this payment was only given to a parent up to when their son or daughter was 16 years of age. This rules out the payment for any full-time carers looking after an adult with an intellectual disability. Many of the carers interviewed expressed frustration at this as they are continuing to do the exact same job.

There were some improvements in the 2004 Budget for those in receipt of Carers Allowance, such as an increase of €10 per week and bringing the weekly income disregard (income not counted as means) to €332.50. In 2009, the maximum weekly rate was €220.50 (for a carer aged under 66, caring for one person).[2] In addition, from 27 September 2007, if carers were getting certain social welfare payments and were providing full time care and attention to another person, they could keep their main social welfare payment and get half-rate Carer's Allowance as well. If a person was getting another social welfare payment before claiming Carer's Allowance, they could get their original payment reinstated and also get half-rate Carer's Allowance.

The carers' groups acknowledged the incremental increases, but maintained it still had a long way to go to access the carers who urgently needed it:

2 Rates available at government website, http://www.welfare.ie.

> At least it is increasing…very slowly each year. Not in line with inflation, but at least it's increasing. And they've had add-ons over the course of time. The television licence fee, the telephone rental, transport pass, electricity units, and the respite grant. They have been added on and it doesn't matter how much of the carers allowance you get, even if you get the lowest, you get all of those in full. That is something but it still has got a huge step to make. (CO2)

The experience of accessing the payments on the ground however gives rise to much frustration for carers. This reflected the gap between the rhetoric regarding its value and the actual level of purpose or use derived from it by carers. Despite recent changes in carers' payments, most were still not entitled to any payment – Carers Allowance or otherwise – that recognised their contribution to society:

> The Carers Allowance is of little or no significance. It applies to very few, a very small percentage of people. And even those who get it, get a reduced amount because of the means testing. (CO2)

The Carer's Allowance is based on traditional notions of family, with a male breadwinner and a female dependent or home-maker. In this case, individualism, which refers to the process by which welfare entitlements are determined on the basis of individual status, rather than a familial one, remains very limited or even deceptive. In the same way, the means-test for carers enquires about the earning level of the spouse; thus policy initiatives and improvements in payments are clearly intended to reinforce the existing model of informal care in the home. This gender ideology frames the eligibility rules for receiving the payment, and in practice, excludes a huge rate of carers from the allowance:

> I don't get full Carer's Allowance because my husband is in the army so I'm means-tested on that. Which I don't approve of. Because my husband goes out working – his wages pays our bills, our mortgage, whatever we have to pay to look after the rest of the family. I mean I have no income for myself. I find that very difficult. (C14)

The failure to abolish the means-test for the Carer's Allowance is a cause of great disappointment to many carers. In practice, a carer will only get the allowance under very stringent conditions, i.e. if they are below the poverty line, have no assets, are unemployed, and often, whether they are married or single. Many carers confirmed this as a reality which was reflected in the low numbers of carers interviewed receiving the payment. In the study, even those who gave up work, either by choice or involuntarily, and were entitled to the payment could not get the full amount as a substitute for lost income;

> I gave up full-time employment. I get a carer's allowance of €46 and 60 pence because of my husband's income. That's what you get. Now... for 48 hours,

> it's not even close to the minimum wage. And I'd say 80 per cent of people get nothing. (C4)

Hence, current social welfare policy ties in strongly with the ideology that women are not perceived as autonomous individuals. The welfare system therefore still tends to support and sustain the patriarchal nuclear family whereby women are treated as dependants of men (Daly, 1989). Despite the support for the nuclear family, in reality there has been little support for women in the home. Most support is provided directly to the breadwinner (by way of dependency allowances). This can be seen as reflecting the patriarchal approach of policy with its reluctance to intervene directly in the family (Cousins, 1995: 42). This fails to recognise the economic argument that it saves the state money by keeping the person in the home instead of a residential care setting:

> It's very unfair on carers – they're talking about it costing 850 Euro per week to keep a person in care. So what's the big thing about paying a carer a proper carer's allowance? Not means-tested. It would be a lot cheaper anyway than putting them in institutions. (C4)

This leads to a more fundamental question as to what essentially is the purpose of the Carer's Allowance in Ireland? Carers typically asked whether it was supposed to be an acknowledgement of their contribution, a community care purchasing method like a direct payment in the UK, or a form of empowerment? In reality, carers thought that it failed to adequately meet any of these needs, and was best understood as a 'token gesture' from the state. Most therefore felt that they were not being adequately recognised. In the first instance, carers certainly felt it did not acknowledge the work they did, as the means-test did not separate the carer's labour from the rest of the family's income:

> At least in England the Carer's Allowance isn't means-tested. You just get it if you're doing the job. I would probably get 18 euros a week – if I was granted a carers allowance. They give other concessions like money off your phone bill. But I mean 18 euro a week? (C21)

Furthermore the payment did not empower the carer or provide a method for purchasing community care, as it failed to perceive them as consumers or clients within the community care system:

> If I had a magic wand, I would give every parent the finances to purchase the services they need. That's the biggest change I would make because, as parents, we're consumers of a service but we don't have the power of a consumer, in that we can't shop around. (C16)

A *Carer's Benefit* was also introduced in October 2000, which requires a record of sufficient social insurance contribution to qualify. This is essentially a payment available for a period of 104 weeks for someone who has given up employment in order to care for someone else. If the care is required for longer than this, the payment terminates, and the carer must enter into the application process for the Carer's Allowance. In reality, it is of little relevance to anyone required to give long-term care. The carers were acutely aware of the time-limit of 104 weeks, and pointed out a range of difficulties with the practicalities of leaving work and applying for the benefit:

> Jeez, my mother lived for 5 years. And what would I have done then? I would have been broke. You know, not only that, but her health was getting worse, and I needed *more* money to look after her. (C21)

At the back of many carers' minds, they also worried that if they took up the benefit, they would not have a job afterwards. Furthermore, from a psychological point of view, some carers spoke about being forced into having a death wish for the person they were looking after, hoping the caring job would be taken out of their hands within the 104 weeks:

> And that's what it is. You're forcing people to actually have a death wish. And not only that; the person then will hang on at their job, they may miss out on it because the person is not going to take a chance. And if they don't live [that long], you say, "oh God, I should have taken that a year beforehand". How do you know? (C16)

In general then, because of these concerns, the Carer's Benefit was a very unpopular social benefit amongst the carers, with many feeling that a fixed time limit excluded this benefit from being of relevance to carers providing long-term care.

More recently, carers are also entitled to an annual *Respite Grant*. The Respite Care Grant is paid once each year, usually in June, for each person a carer is caring for. This grant increased from €835 in 2004 to €1,700 in June 2009.[3] However, in the experience of the carer organisations interviewed, the means-test still excludes most. Furthermore, all the grants and allowances are subject to different eligibility rule changes with each annual budget, as illustrated by the following carer:

> Well, I have to say now, up to last year, I did get the Respite Grant. I don't know what happened this year. I'm even afraid to ask. (C14)

Carers and disabled people alike are thus always in a position of powerless dependency on budget fluctuations and political decisions. What might be available one year may be curtailed the next, and if another excluded group becomes

3 Rates available at http://www.citizensinformation.ie.

'popular' in mainstream society, the fixed resources must be fought for among the other dependent groups, in effect robbing one to feed the other. It is important to understand therefore that with statutory care, it also means an acceptance of control (see Close, 1995). When having a disabled child or relative that needs to be cared for in a household the carer must enter into a discourse, albeit a one-sided one with the state.

Accessing the 'Health Services'

The health services are generally the access point to most community care services at the regional level, even though many of these services are delivered by the non-profit sector. The health services provide a diverse array of supports such as information, home-help attendants, general practitioners, and social services much like having the combined roles of the NHS and local authorities in the UK. The health services are divided into three sectors: general hospital and primary care; special hospital care; and community care. Spending on community-based services for people with disabilities amounted to an estimated €1.5 billion in 2007 (Inclusion Ireland, 2010).

Despite the transition from health boards to Health Service Executives, which saw a decrease in regional bodies from 11 to 4 (see Comptroller and Auditor General, 2008), many critics have argued that this is purely a cosmetic change. This is argued as being due to the resistance by health boards to rationalise their organisation and cut duplication, because real reform will most likely mean job cuts in administration. The position adopted by the Government in the 10 year National Health Strategy (2001) also raised serious questions in light of the latest health reports. In the Strategy, the Government said that while the number of health boards should be subject to review, it had 'carefully considered whether the current number [previously 11 regional bodies] best meets the requirements of the health system. It is satisfied that changing the number of health boards would not of itself lead to improvements in services.' (Bowers, 2005).

While this may be true, the national carer organisations, which are in regular contact with each regional Health Board, were acutely aware of the regional variation in coverage between Health Board regions of carer services across Ireland. According to the Carer's Association, carer support varies regionally, depending upon the efficiency, priorities and structuring of the health boards and the coverage of the voluntary sector, thus leading to geographical differences in levels of support:

> It completely depends on Health Boards. There is a huge amount of inconsistency. We could bring you to take families living only a couple of miles from each other with the River Shannon in the middle. And the River Shannon seems to have a huge effect on services between various different health boards. I mean it's not just between [Western] Health Boards and other ones. It's all over the

place. And you will find like, I can think of Health Boards off the top of my head and I can say to myself, 'well, if I was a carer and I was looking after a child with a disability I would definitely like to be living in X'. I might want to be in a different health board, in a different part of the country. And I think that can depend an awful lot on personalities within health boards. (CO1)

Much of this difference stems from the different staff divisions in each Health Board. Under the umbrella of Community Care many different positions exist – from carer co-ordinators to home-help co-ordinators – and each Health Board is responsible for how it sets up these posts. This leads to much regional differentiation in how community care is delivered:

There are health board areas that have carer co-ordinators, and there are those that don't, and I think that would be interesting to look at because I think some of the carer co-ordinators are very effective – I think it can be an enormous benefit. And the health boards that don't have them, maybe carers are at a disadvantage there. (CO1)

For instance, according to the Midland Health Board Annual Report (2004), links with the Carers Association are very strong in the Longford/Westmeath Community Care Areas, where the carer co-ordinator works with this organisation on the recruitment of carers for the training programme, the facilitation of information days and running carer clinics across the two counties.

Carers are also very conscious of the geographic differences across health boards of rights to services. In particular are those who participate in voluntary work themselves. It was argued by participants that different health boards had different policies regarding care; hence having a significant influencing effect in the way caring was dealt with. The experiences of carers and those cared for were affected by variations in the availability and ease of accessing particular resources. Thus the findings suggest that carer's experiences of their local space varies according to the different social, medical, and political relations within the jurisdictional climate of their local health board:

The [East] health board seem to look after their carers an awful lot better than they do up this side. I mean all those Carer's weekends away, I pay for all my weekends, when they're all funded to go. If you go down and represent [County A] at a meeting, you pay your own way. Whereas the [North] Health Board subsidise it. And they have their own fundraising thing on the side as well. (C4)

If Nicola was born now down in [County A], from the time she was born, she would have been handed a medical card. There and then. Because she's Down's Syndrome; Medical Card automatically. Because my brother's son was born

> within six weeks of Nicola, and he had Down's Syndrome as well. Now the fact that he was born in [County B], you don't get a Medical Card. (C21)

In examining methods of welfare allocation, such as this, the issues of social justice and rights, as discussed in Chapter 3, are of key concern at the local scale. The equitable access to resources and the benefits derived from social rights are more apparent at this scale, where the actual mechanisms behind resource distribution decisions are clearer (Meade and Earickson, 2000). In most cases, political parties have developed a range of cost-control strategies as a way of rationing such services. Often, these involve control measures to be put in place to avert crisis away from them, as ambitious political agendas come into conflict with tight budgetary constraints (Kane, 1997). While bureaucracy is a necessary part of government administration, often government is criticised by its tendency to concentrate authority in a complex structure of administration, characterised by routine, insistence on forms ('red tape') and regulations, with a hierarchy of bureaus and agencies, thus forming a large, complex and cumbersome administrative structure (Wilson 1982).

This situation raises the question as to whether the community care services act in the interests of their clients, or just in their own interest, to maintain the appearance of a comprehensive care system. Age Action argued that the overall community care system, for elderly and disabled alike, works simply to its own needs:

> I think the services are not there to meet the needs of the community, of the carer, or the person they are caring for. It's slow, it's cumbersome, it doesn't operate to the needs of the carer, it operates to the needs of the system. The system operates it, not the patients. So it's the system working for the system, not for the people. (CO4)

One of the first major problems with the administration of community care services is the reliance on local Teachta Dáila's (TDs) (local government councillors who also have a seat in national parliament) at the Health Board level. This is a legacy of Ireland's corporatist governance structure, where contacting local political representatives is still a common occurrence for many carers. As discussed in Chapter 3, government constraints on health and welfare expenditure mean that they cannot provide all the care a State might wish to and therefore decisions have to be made about the nature and range of services to provide. These are questions of a geographical, as well as an economic, political, and managerial nature, since such services will have to be provided some*where* (Gatrell, 2002). In Ireland's case, local political representatives often play gatekeepers and arrange the allocation of services:

> I spoke to a carer in one of our services not long ago and he had been quite a political animal when he was a younger man, and he's the first person, no matter what happens with his wife, if there is anything he needs, he rings his TD. (CO5)

This focus on the local political agent aggravates many of the carers interviewed and voluntary organisations alike. While many parents were forced to access their services through this means, they fundamentally disagreed with the fairness of this method of delivering services:

> It's just the way it works. People say we haven't got a good TD for our area. There's no point in voting for him because he won't do anything for you, rather than looking at the whole country, and saying, "we all live in this bloody island, and a Down's Syndrome child shouldn't be treated any different in [Stamullen] than in [Skerries]". But they are. (C21)

There is therefore a strong need to standardise services across the health boards, instead of relying on political favours at local level. As discussed, social rights, in contrast to civil and political rights, are largely viewed as political programmes, and are depicted as involving high levels of state expenditure and intervention. It therefore becomes an issue of whom the state values more rather than social justice. Although voluntary organisations advocate a change in the system, from one based on who you know and how loud you shout, to one offering a fairer allocation of resources, many still felt compelled to advise carers to 'play the game' as it was:

> I have talked to families who ring their TD just to try and get their placement! This is what we tell people to do. In one way, you feel like you're contributing to a system that's already not fair, and it's terribly problematic because if we encourage them to do it, then they get prioritised over somebody else. That's how it is. And then you've got all the other people who don't know, who never heard of [Inclusion Ireland], or say, "Oh I suppose I'll have to put up with it". (CO6)

This scenario, in combination with resource issues, has led to excessive waiting lists for community services. This is most clearly seen in the problems associated with ordering equipment from health boards. The experience of ordering essential aids such as walking supports for people with Down's Syndrome, or wheelchairs for those with multiple-impairments causes a great deal of frustration due to excessive waiting lists:

> When you want something, you want it then. Particularly with [Pauline] because she's mentally handicapped and if she breaks something, or something goes wrong, she needs it within nearly 24 hours. But you wait 6 months for the Health Board to get anything. (C19)

To compound this problem, carers are not allowed to order any equipment to accommodate for impending needs under a future service plan. Instead, calls for equipment can only be made when the need arises. One carer was acutely aware of the rationing that goes on at this level, in relation to the allocation of equipment. When asked about whether they had to pay for their equipment themselves, one carer argued that they: *"put you under terrible pressure. You've got this aid, so now you've got your quota for the year"* (C19).

Ideally, trained professionals would support carers through the delicate process of determining rights and services, but often this relationship is difficult as professionals regularly do not have a very good understanding of the families' point of view and their experiences (Jones, 2002: 159). In the interviews, for example, when those carers interviewed got information and advice from clinicians, it was often limiting, and limited the potential of the person with the disability:

> I found that from the professionals, while they were good, they always put ceilings on their advice. And any ambition you would have for your child to do things, they always said, "remember he has Down's Syndrome; don't expect him to do this, don't expect him to do that". And I found it very depressing. (C16)

As discussed earlier, the transition period immediately following the end of their formal schooling can be highly stressful for young adults with intellectual disabilities and their parents. The difficulty of this transition is exacerbated by experiences such as this, where the families are faced with non-supportive interactions. These are defined as unhelpful interactions and behaviours that occur in relationships which are designed as sources of support, yet have a disproportionate negative influence on psychological health (Neufeld et al., 2007). Drawing on these general experiences with dealing with the health services, the following section explores the experiences of carers of the interventions of the main agents within the health services' community care system; social workers, public health nurses, and home-helps.

Social Workers and Public Health Nurses

Personal social services are the responsibility of the health services. However, historically social services in Ireland largely focused primarily on children, adults as parents, and child protection. Debates on social work in relation to other groups such as people with disabilities are largely absent (Powell, 1998). Walsh (1999) describes how the state, the Catholic Church, and the medical profession actively resisted the development of professional social work services in Ireland. The establishment of unified social service departments in the UK is contrasted with the more reactive and piecemeal development of social work in Ireland.

The need for the intervention of a social worker is crucial at the time when a care recipient is facing adulthood. The carers interviewed seemed to lack specific knowledge about services after school. They experienced less opportunity than normal to meet other parents at the start and end of the school day. One carer in particular was going through this transition, at the time of the study, and demonstrates that parent's sometimes have a reluctance to seek out information because by doing so they must face very stressful concerns about the future:

> My biggest worry is that [Jenny] is 18 now, she leaves school and where am I going to get services? She gets physio in school in the CRC. She gets all her services there. Where am I going to go? It's going to be very fragmented. And I say to my husband, 'what are we going to do?' And he just says, 'we'll wait and see'. But what is going to happen is if Lindsey needs physio, we're going to have to pay. I mean, she gets her disability allowance. That's going to pay for her physio, so she's not going to ever be able to save money for her future. We're trying to put it by for her. (C14)

One of the main gaps which carers spoke of was proper support at this vital period. The difficulty in accessing information has obvious implications for carers trying to act as an advocate for their adult son or daughter in accessing services. The importance of early intervention is illustrated very well by one carer who said, *"the secret with any medical problem, or whatever condition, is early recognition of the problem. And early intervention" (C21)*. However many have negative experiences in this regard:

> [Carers] are not put in touch with the social worker or the public health nurse, and nobody seems to have the responsibility for backing up the family and guiding them and taking them through what's going to be a very long process. (CO5)

When asked what the main service gaps were, some carers talked about the general lack of services across the spectrum:

> All over. Right from the very beginning. I've seen it operating for 25 years and it hasn't changed in that 25 years; in neither its attitude to the ability of people with DS, or in its service that it provides. All you need, as I said, is support and someone to say to you, "we're doing the best we can, we will try this, we will have this". Not closed minds. I've had 25 years experience and I know; I've tried different things to get there. (C24)

Carers found it very difficult to access information on what services were available, who provides them, how they qualified for them, and whether they were available in their area. Of all the tasks that carers had to face, finding information about services, resources, and sources of support for care recipients and themselves was one of the most daunting. It appeared to them that services are fragmented and getting the information about support options was one of the key challenges for the future sustainability of the community care system. Carers often had to find their way around many gatekeepers and eligibility concerns, in order to constantly maintain their knowledge of available supports. In reality though, carers had great difficulty keeping up to date with changes in legislation, their rights entitlements, and how the system is administered, and without a comprehensive needs assessment some of the carers went without services they were eligible for. In one instance, a carer had the household's garage converted for the care recipient to live independently, only to find out later there was a grant for house conversion from the local authorities. More generally, carers argued that the information deficit felt like a smoke-screen for the service users, thus suggesting the gap between the aims of ambitious political programs and the resource constraints:

> There's nothing. There's supposed to be social workers but they don't really tell you anything either. They told us nothing. Anything we have, or did, we did it ourselves. By ringing or the internet. Talking to people. That's how we found out practically everything. It's almost like a smokescreen. There are services there but nobody tells you […] There's not that much you can do. You can't fight the system, you're just at their mercy really. (C3)

Carers normally have to go through a period of acceptance where the long-term nature of the change in their life is acknowledged, alongside an emerging understanding that they are likely to continue to need support over a long-term period (Jones, 2002). Often parents cling to a hope for quite a lengthy period that the disability or illness can be cured. This difficulty in *accepting* the long-term nature of the problem is agitated by the difficulty in obtaining information which could alleviate much of the worrying. For carers, this results in a constant battling with health boards and practitioners, that becomes a fundamental aspect of life as a carer:

> That's the way you find things out – if you weren't the type of person who wanted this contact with other people, you're just left. I was just left with him here. And I kept ringing [the Health Board] up... and I just tormented them. (C3)

According to *Care Alliance*, discovering who should be contacted, what should be asked, and what one is entitled to, is very difficult. This has knock-on effects for many carers, especially those who may be less vocal about their rights. In the interviews with carers, many admitted resorting to finding out everything on their own:

> There was nothing. I just read these books and got more and more depressed, and was just trying to carry on as best I could. (C7)

> I had to find out everything myself. It's just not out there in front of you. You have to go rooting for it, and you have to find out everything. There's no need's assessment. (C14)

In a lot of cases, information about eligibility for certain benefits or about a parents' support group, came through unofficial channels. For instance, some carers found out about services through chance encounters with parents in the same situation. Therefore, as well as reading books, carers cited informal sources of information as a crucial way of finding out important data about the disability, and what help was available:

> You're very much on your own really. As I said the biggest help I got was from fellow parents who are either going through it or have gone through it. And that's where you get all your help. (C8)

Many carers reported finding themselves banging against a brick wall most of the time in terms of accessing formal sources of information. When asked for their experiences of dealing with health boards for information, carers gave primarily negative responses:

> [If] you ring up, and say you're enquiring, they'll say, "well hold on, I'll put you through to this". And then you get through to this one, and you've to go to another one. There should be someone there who can tell you. (C14)

> You get no reply letter from any letter that you write. You're wasting your time. I mean, the Health Boards don't even inform you of what's available. (C4)

Part of the problem stems from the fact that there is no formal needs-assessment and care plan made out for the carer when the child turns 18. There are well-defined health, educational and social needs of a person growing up with an intellectual disability and with proper early-intervention, many families could cope much better without the undue stress of having to find out these things too late. Some carers, for example, reported not being told about known health problems associated with Down's Syndrome:

> I had no idea [children with down's syndrome] are more prone to colds and ear infections. I was never told that. Because in the end (Paul's) ears became so bad, he had to get a hearing aid. (C5)

Although the government has indicated person-centred planning in recent policy, in reality the delivery of services has been seen as knee-jerk reactions to crises:

> the only way to get the health system to react in my experience would be when a crisis arises. And that's the only time when a bed will suddenly be found, or the PHN will come out, or whatever it is. Or like, that something will move and shake in the system out of nowhere. I mean if you're in dire straits, you will get a social-worker. They certainly aren't there to enable people or empower people. Which I think would be wonderful. (C16)

Therefore when asked whether carers had received help from a social worker, through a needs assessment, they generally expressed their disappointment with the lack of provision:

> There was nobody coming and offering anything. I never saw a social-worker, apart from the one who was part of the early intervention team, I have never actually had a social-worker who came to see how he was getting on, or what's he doing or anything like that. (C16)

The public health nurse is another vital link in the community care chain. Although community care comes under the remit of the public health nurses, in practice the work load consisting of administering public health vaccines, aiding older people and new babies, means that carers and adults with intellectual disabilities are largely beyond the resources and time available to the nurses:

> The PHN in this area, I'd say the woman has that much work to do already. Between all the new babies and the unmarried mothers, and the older people, and the school injections. I don't think it would be fair. I think there should be two on duty, no one person can cover the radius that woman has to cover. I mean she should have a younger nurse with her to do the babies, or the old people, whichever takes the most work. They don't even have proper help. (C4)

Therefore, public health nurses have very little contact with the carers in their jurisdiction. Again, the problem of too much rigidity in the administration came up in relation to public health nurses:

> There's a problem of professions being stuck in their box as well – there's no co-ordination at all. (C16)

This is an inevitable outcome of the decline in generic services in community care. The rise in professional specialisation of front-line staff however, has meant a deterioration in communication between the new specialised clinicians and front-line workers within the community care spectrum.:

> Well there is the whole rig-ma-role with people only being able to do certain things…But there aren't enough Occupational Therapists, Public Health Nurses, or physiotherapists within the community to serve the needs of today. They are serving certain needs for yesterday, many yesterday's past. When they are turning up today, they will have been needed 18 months ago. So it's the system working for the system, not for the people. (CO6)

Respite: Home-Help Attendants

Respite refers to a temporary interval of rest or relief provided to people with disabilities or their caregivers in order that their families can take a break from the daily routine of caregiving. This is to help prevent physical and mental exhaustion, and support family unity. Traditionally, respite generally was conceived of as a break which enabled family members to take holidays, or just a few hours of time off. In practice, respite comes in two forms; firstly, 'in-home' respite refers to respite programs which send a formal carer, or home-help attendant, to the family's home, and secondly; 'day-care' respite which means the individual with the disability goes to a day care centre or 'respite placement', with an emphasis on relieving the caregiver (discussed in the next Respite Centres section). This is generally, although not exclusively, provided by the health services. Respite is quite different to residential long-term care in its ethos; it is still focused on keeping people within the community for as long as possible.

Ireland's approach to temporary domiciliary support began with the home help service, which was established as a statutory service under Section 65 of the *Health Act* (1970). Under the Act, health boards are empowered (not obliged) to provide a discretionary home help service for sick or infirm people or their dependents, women who have recently given birth and people who would otherwise need institutional care. In practice, older people constitute the largest category of clients of the service (O'Donovan, 1997). In terms of geographical access, the criteria for eligibility varies from one region to the next, as the existence of support from family frequently disqualifies people from eligibility (Ruddle, 1994). Therefore the presence of informal carers means that they may not be able to access home help support services.

The home help service provides an example of the lack of commitment to resourcing community-based services in Ireland. Instead of providing training, it is clear when considering the nature of the care provided by home helps, that the health services consider home-help as non-technical work, maintaining that it is a form of paid-volunteering in nature. This is reflected in the rates of pay for home helps, where payments are symbolic and unrelated to market levels of wages (O'Donovan, 1997). According to the community care manager of one of the health service executive areas, they provide a supervisory role, and rely on low-skilled and generally low paid 'volunteer' workers within the non-profit sector:

> You can basically say that the home help service is provided on a voluntary basis. In that there are committees throughout the whole '[Northern] Area region' that we fund through what we call Section 65 grants. So what basically happens is there are local committees and they come to us and look for money. And what we do is employ the organiser, and then they go out and recruit home helps on our behalf…So we would fund them and pay one supervisor to make sure the work is being done. (HSEA Respondent 1)

However, at the time of the this study, home-help hours had been cut in half by one of the HSEA's. As anticipated, many carers were incensed by this, feeling that cutting a programme in this way was thoughtless and nearsighted. Home-help funding is not ring-fenced by the health services, and is thus susceptible to erratic annual changes in funding:

> They're so bloody mean about the service. It used to be 5 hours; it's 3 now. So it was just a short break to go into town. It's a very short time to do anything with. That's a big cut-back. It's all cut-backs, cut-backs. And for them, it's just really statistics really – they look at the figures. (C17)

> The 10 hours of home-help was brilliant but now with the 5 hours, I don't get anytime to myself. I mean I am not getting any younger. I'm getting on and I get very tired. (C14)

Although home help is looked upon as the keystone of community care, if not funded properly, many carers felt it was of little use. However, despite the many frustrations carers felt with the home help service, Care Alliance advocated that carers safeguard their few hours of home help a week:

> if you have it or if you can get it, you hang on to it because if it goes it's very hard to get it back. It's very hard to get into the system – either the home help or respite. You know, you take what you can get, not necessarily what you need or what you want. (CO2)

Respite Centres

The other form of respite available is 'day-care' respite which means the individual with the disability goes to a day care centre or 'respite placement', with an emphasis on relieving the caregiver. As mentioned previously, this is to provide a temporary interval of rest or relief to people with disabilities or their caregivers in order that their families can take a break from the daily routine of caregiving. However, in contrast to home-help or other forms of domicilliary attendant care, the idea of 'day-care' respite as a period of time when the stress and responsibility of caregiving is temporarily transferred to trained providers so that the carer may enjoy that time with peace of mind has come under much scrutiny recently. Many people with disabilities have resisted this notion and, perhaps in echoing their concerns, it has become quite contested within the literature (see Chappell et al., 2001). On the one hand, this form of respite has promoted the notion that the care recipient is a source of burden and should be removed from the home, with an acceptance that caregivers can relinquish responsibility to someone they do not know. This is particularly the case with many forms of day-care respite. This is aggravated by the majority of research which tends to assume that caregiving creates burden and decreases well-being, rather than something that can be simultaneously experienced with well-being (see Yates et al., 1999; Chappell and Reid, 2002).

On the other hand, the reality is respite *can be* a valuable service to carers and can prevent caregiver breakdown and delaying placement of the care recipient in long-term care (Canadian Association for Community Care, 1998; Kosloski and Montgomery, 1995). Indeed, respite is one of the most frequently expressed needs of caregivers (Wykle, 1994), although the term itself need not be familiar to many caregivers who speak of needing a break.

The carers in this study acknowledged how useful it was to get a few hours of freedom during the day. For many, this is the only opportunity to get away from the home. This is important given that research (see Acton, 2002) has shown that many caregivers do not have the time to engage in health-promoting self-care. Acton also found that the likelihood of engaging in self-care is influenced by individual characteristics (age, gender, culture, education, income, and stress levels) and values of certain self-care behaviours (perceived importance of self-care, barriers, and ability to implement self-care strategies). The study concluded that caregivers practice fewer self-care behaviours than other non-caregivers. Those who were able to practice self-care experienced lower levels of stress and the effects of stress on their wellbeing.

In terms of respite within the health services, the carers interviewed felt that there were not enough respite centres. There are significant variations between the health boards with the highest number of places and attendance's found in the Western Health Board and the lowest number found in the South Western Health Board. There were 395,868 attendance's at respite centres overall (National Disability Authority, 2004: 70). Although official numbers seem small, the majority of these cases are those where families have been experiencing extreme stress, often for periods of years, attempting to cope in frequently intolerable conditions (Merriman and Canavan, 2007). Waiting lists continue to grow in part as a result of the changing age profile of people with intellectual disabilities. The birth rate in the 1960s and 1970s has resulted in a cohort of adults in their 20s and 30s requiring full-time residential services, whilst people with an intellectual disability are living longer and using services more (National Disability Authority, 2004: 53). According to one carer organisation, this means there are considerable waiting lists for the centres that operate:

> People who need to book a holiday, or take a break, they have to book about 6 to 8 months in advance. I've known people through the helpline who've told me that, "they've been told they haven't got a chance". Now how can you plan with that? (CO6)

Carers felt that respite on the ground was insufficiently funded to cater for their needs. They were of the opinion that the demand for the service completely outweighed the supply. Moreover, by acknowledging the difficulty of the job, many felt it had to be suitably funded:

> They seem to have money for every other department but there doesn't seem to be anything there for respite care or for health regards mentally handicapped people, nor for the facilities even to pay the staff properly. That's why they cannot get caring staff. If they paid the right money, they'd get the right staff. I mean that's the hardest job out there. Who else would do it? (C4)

As a consequence of the restrictions on respite places and the difficulty gaining access, many felt vulnerable as a result of this service gap. In particular, many families who did not have other natural supports felt isolated, because in many cases, there was no back-up available in case of an accident except for the emergency services. According to one carer, this feeling of isolation was more pronounced during the afternoon, when neighbours were working:

> Even say, the likes of me; I'm only a carer. If anything goes wrong with Sharon, I may ring the emergency services. I've nobody here. I'm in the middle of the country. Where would you get anyone around here all day – they're all working. Everybody is working. I guarantee you can knock at every door the whole way from this house to Maynooth, and you will not get one woman home. And I wouldn't know that only a man selling fire-extinguishers came and he told me you're the only woman each side of the road, from Maynooth the whole way out. And that's five mile each side of the road. Everybody's working he said. (C4)

To highlight the other side of the debate regarding the suitability of respite as an option however, parents acknowledged that their adult child with an intellectual disability can find it difficult to deal with the transition to a respite centre. Many people with an intellectual disability feel uncomfortable, nervous, or confused with the change in care setting. It appeared that most carers were aware of the dislike felt by their child towards such an option. In particular, one carer argued that:

> We had a lot of problems with [respite care] because he did not like this.... being with all the other handicapped children…because he was used to an environment where he had only one brother and he was free to do whatever he wanted (C2).

Some parents find it difficult to communicate the idea of a temporary break away from home in a respite centre to the person. According to one of the care agencies, who themselves provide respite, the transition to a respite place can be quite distressing for a young adult with intellectual disabilities:

> They are totally discommoded. Their room is different, where they eat is different, even the plates they eat on are quite different. (CO3)

Part of this problem is the presumption made by many service providers of a respite 'place' being very limited, and often meaning a bed in a room. By right, some service providers are aware of these limitations, yet are restricted in what they can provide. Very often, there are no extra resources for the facility to make the stay more comfortable for the person with the disability. According to one carer who was reluctant to use the respite options available:

> You see a lot of problems we're having is they're buying these day centres and they put the blocks there but they forget the equipment. They give the grants for the block work. But there's nothing else. And that's where the real expenses come. It's all a fight then when it comes to that. (C19)

Despite waiting lists, generally if the 'place' in the centre is being filled, the health services are happy that the service corresponds to the demand. However, in reality the carers' negative reactions to the respite centres suggest that the service once again works for the service, not for the clients, in that there is limited flexibility in meeting the preferences of the service-users. Although it is a service for people with disabilities, again there is the expectation that the person does not have any behavioural problems, extra impairments or health problems even though incongruously it is the carers of these people that need a break the most:

> It depends again – if your child is very good, you will get respite. If your child has diabetes and a heart condition, you won't get respite. (C16)

> Well you don't want to just dump her with someone. That you have a great weekend, and she's a miserable one. What good is that? Respite is in its infancy. And respite is looked at like, 'yeah, we have a bed in a room, and food'. (C21)

As a result, although a few of the carers interviewed used respite, the majority of carers talked about their fears of leaving their son or daughter in the types of care settings that are available. In response to the conflicts over the appropriateness of respite, the notion of respite *as an outcome* rather than *as a service*, encourages a fundamental shift in the way we understand the concept and practice of respite. Rather than viewing respite simply as a service to caregivers, it should be seen more appropriately as an outcome for caregivers. This opens the idea of respite up to a much wider conceptualisation of supports for the person with the disability incorporating a range of options such as finding work, volunteering, community groups, sports clubs, painting classes, etc. This is the converse of respite *as a service*, which describes the much narrower respite options mentioned above. These are thought to offer a 'quick fix' of symptoms, rather than addressing the cause. According to Chappell (2001), even when respite services (in the traditional sense) are utilised, it is not at all clear that they are effective; citing several studies which report little or no effect of these programmes (Opie et al., 1992 in New Zealand; Milne et al., 1993 in Great Britain; Nolan et al., 1993 in the United

States). Many reasons have been put forward for this, including unfamiliarity, cost, psychosocial conflicts over the appropriateness of respite care; philosophical values opposed to respite care; fear of loss of independence; lack of understanding of bureaucratic structures; and negative attitudes towards the receipt of services. Hartrick (1997) supports moving beyond a service model of respite that works as a 'quick fix', to a practice that supports building the capacity of families, transforms relationships and discovers new sources of support.

As an alternative to 'day-care' respite models, some carers advocated setting up more structured natural sources of care, from neighbours and friends. Choosing to have an au-pair or some other form of care assistance in the home also appeared to be a more satisfactory solution for carers, as opposed to formal care outside the home. Like in the UK care model where you can employ someone who is comfortable and well-used to the person, carers saw the benefit in being able to hire someone privately:

> In reality what you need to do is develop extended families as such. For example, if someone had a friendship or relationship with [Claire], and found it comfortable to come over, and [Claire] found it comfortable to go to them. So they're looked upon as a visitor or friend. And I think that's the model to develop. (C21)

This informal care option being advocated echoes recent trends elsewhere towards developing natural connections within the community. One such example is the community connector models being developing in British Columbia, Canada, such as Vela Microboards and the Planned Lifetime Advocacy Network. These aim to develop relationships with people within the community based on a persons' wishes and goals. Furthermore, these models advocate moving away from the idea of respite as an entitlement towards developing options which allow respite as an outcome to be achieved.

Accessing the Non-profit Sector Services

In accordance to the subsidiarity principle, the government has maintained that its role (through the health authorities) be limited to providing clinical services, some respite, and financial assistance to voluntary bodies. As a result, the voluntary or non-profit sector is generally the next point of call after a young adult leaves school for most families. As discussed in the last chapter, the voluntary sector has an extensive coverage of intellectual disability services across Ireland. Due to the lack of prior statutory coverage of community care services historically, the health services have targeted non-profit organisations as well as local voluntary groups, such as meals-on-wheels. These non-profit organisations provide a wide spectrum of supports from residential provision, transport, day services and supported employment. As discussed, in certain areas the sector has also been funded to provide such things as a home help service and information clinics. In 2004, the former health boards and the former Eastern Regional Health Authority (ERHA) collectively paid €877m to nonprofit organisations providing services to disabled persons (C&AG, 2005). Most voluntary organisations now have close partnership relationships with the state, often depending on statutory funding for survival.

At the same time, as the last chapter identified, fund-raising is still a substantial part of some non-profit agencies' funding. Even some organisations providing essential services for people with intellectual disabilities must rely on their own fund-raising. *Down Syndrome Ireland* is a primary example; it provides family support, social and education services for people with Down's Syndrome, encourages research and disseminates information; and improves public awareness and knowledge of Down's Syndrome. At the local level however, a large portion of funding for the organisation's branches comes from fundraising. A lot of the parents are actively involved themselves in the fund-raising activities:

> Em…it's recognised as an issue more. Yes. People are highlighting it more all the time. It's in the media. But actually on the ground, the improvements are very difficult to see. If you take our own business here, Down's Syndrome Ireland; speech therapy, music therapy and an early intervention. And all of that we have to provide through fund-raising. So it does mean, we're out on a limb; all the time, we're out there fund-raising. And it means long-term planning is very difficult. It means it's very fragmented across scale. (C16)

While this compounds the issue of the sector's relative independence from the state, in reality, the majority of providers receive their funding from government in the broader area of service provision. Thus while there has been a huge commitment to altruism and mutualism in Ireland historically, with the State adopting a hands-off approach as identified earlier, for the most part, the Health Service Executives have responsibility for administering block grants to nonprofit organisations in their regional areas. Since then, allocations have been made by means of a global grant to the directly funded agencies on the basis of the previous year's outturn, which in turn was based on the outturn of the year before that. Allocations are also made on the basis of proposals to improve or expand services, and the availability of finance generally (Ryan, 1999). There is typically little connection between the size of the grant and the numbers cared for, the category of disability or the degree of disability. Critics note that the manner in which funding is released seems to militate against forward planning (Donoghue, 2002).

In terms of how the non-profit sector appears on the ground, the family care associations interviewed were very aware of these broader policy climate issues. According to one agency, this loose funding system led to much regional disparity across health service regions. This was typified by the means with which health boards fund and allocate tasks to the voluntary organisations. In some areas, there was an obvious commitment to provide community services formally, through the health services, instead of through the use of non-profit agencies:

> Well I know definitely the [North] Health Board is progressive in the sense that it itself provides a lot of the services, rather than having the voluntary organisations doing it for them, and the services that they do provide are very professional in the sense that they develop self-advocacy and they're really moving on things. (CO3)

On the other hand, in areas where a Health Board is deemed to be less progressive, the voluntary sector has, perhaps by necessity over time, become a much stronger provider of services and advocate:

> You have the [West] Health Board who has two or three residential services who would provide for a couple of hundred people. And their services are dire. I mean some of them are the worst in the country. And again because there is no funding prioritised, the Health Board are plodding along, while you have voluntary organisations in the same Health Board area doing wonderful things. (CO3)

This situation is likely to have arisen in areas where there were large residential institutions inherited from the Victorian era, and where community care was developed solely by parent and friends associations. These costly institutions have remained part of the landscape of care due to the high transition costs associated with moving people back into the community and are currently being funded by the health services. As a result, these Health Service Executive areas must rely on the non-profit sector for providing a community service. The following sections examine in more detail the core service options for young adults with intellectual disabilities provided by the non-profit sector.

Adult Day Services

Adult day services make up the most significant portion of the support options for young adults with intellectual disabilities. In Ireland, as identified, the non-profit sector provides the majority of day services in the community. These cover a wide range of options such as sheltered workshops, day support, and occupational training (discussed in the next section).

Despite the successes which the sector has achieved in being able to target the needs of different impairments directly, these successes in and of themselves have created a number of challenges. Over time, as a result of the loose formal contracting or tendering process, the service catchments of many providers have became more decentralised and inconsistent, responding to localised needs, or being prompted differently by active individuals. In these cases, it appeared that the care service often operates to meet its own ends, and not for the interests of the users.

> Well [Michael] is 24 now and I suppose the onus is on the family despite all the services that appear to be there on paper. If you don't slot into their box, it's quite bureaucratic. And it's either a take it or leave it scenario. While they all talk about Person Centred Planning, and they all talk the talk, when you actually go to look for a service, if you're not within their service, if what you want is not in their service, just forget it. It's actually a waste of time. (C15)

While 'person-centred planning' was often used in the rhetoric of service providers, carers often felt they were dealing with a mechanistic organisation, with a conservative ethos, more concerned with the internal work of meeting the present needs of the organisation, than responding to their needs and helping them. According to Osbourne (1998), these traits are characteristic of bureaucratic organisations, which are formalised, and more suitable for stable conditions than ones requiring flexibility.

While Powell and Guerin (1997: 11) argue that the voluntary sector is perceived as an alternative to State bureaucracy and professional elitism, in Ireland the complicated service relationship between State and voluntary sectors can often lead to even greater bureaucracy. According to the interviews, carers were very accustomed to dealing with 'red tape' in accessing such services. On the whole, both carers and advocacy bodies thought services geared towards supporting community care were in reality largely cosmetic on the ground.

Many carers felt that day services were characterised as being overly regimental and stringent. Therefore there is little room for people not fitting into clear administrative categories to gain services. This has profound implications for those whose particular disability doesn't 'fit' the service providers remit. For example, when the person has behavioural problems, this adds to the difficulty in finding a day support provider willing to offer a place. The following quote is from a family who had great difficulty in accessing a service provider and in the end had to accept a poor fit of service:

> We applied to [St Pauls] and…they weren't too keen on taking him because he hadn't got Down's Syndrome. And they were saying we could put him out in the ordinary school. We stood up and said. 'you couldn't put him into a normal school'. He couldn't speak. They taught him sign-language. Prior to that, he was like an explosive bomb. It was terrible. So in the end they took him. They didn't really want to take him. And what do you do if they say we don't want to take him? – keep him at home? Send him to a school and they'd ring you up and say, 'take him out of here please'. (C4)

As the above quote demonstrates, the 'goodness-of-fit' between the current menu of service options and the needs of individuals with a disability is, at times, questionable. For example, carers found an implicit expectation that their adult child does not have any behavioural problems, extra impairments or health problems. Ironically, as disclosed by most families, it is these individuals and their carers that need the most help. This leaves parents in a position where they often must consider services which are inappropriate to the needs of their son or daughter, and which may not fully develop their potential. Furthermore, it also means that the unique expertise which parents possess about their own children is not being capitalised upon at a vital time of decision making (Redmond, 1996: 37).

When families were successful in getting their child a place in a day service, generally the level of satisfaction varied depending on the level of expectation of the parents, as well as the ability level of the individual. In many cases, carers found the activities offered by their day centre as quite positive:

> Yes, he's quite happy, because here at the [care] centre we have pottery classes, and Thursday night we have drawing and they all have special needs. And they enjoy coming and meeting and joining up with their friends. (C17)

However, it was obvious that other carers had a much higher level of expectation from their service; particularly around independence training and finding a job. In these cases, the parents felt that their service was less well equipped to deal with these demands. Some compared them to custodial centres with little meaningful activity:

> Now she's in the day centre. Day centres are very bad. They're very badly equipped. They go into the day centres and sit there all day. There's not much activity there for them. For the likes of [Mary] there isn't, because she can't really do much. But you'd think they'd take them out somewhere. Even out shopping. (C16)

Part of the problem is the wide differences in learning difficulty within the intellectual disability spectrum, making it very difficult to cater for everyone. There was some evidence from the interviews with service providers of tailoring services to particular levels of individuals' ability. One provider in particular was trying to provide for the person's needs by means of a 'facilitator', instead of a 'trainer'. This means that the person with the disability has greater say in their own well-being and identifying their needs, instead of having to do a fixed course for everyone, regardless of impairment. According to one parent of a child using this provider:

> At the moment he's doing what they call a self-advocacy course. And I think according to their ability, some of them are doing computers, you know, so... to get them jobs is the difficult thing – for anybody with a disability. But I'd hope he will because he's certainly well-capable. Even something for say, 2 hours a day? Just to get out of the house. (C7)

On the other hand, because of the varying degree of 'fit' between a service provider's supports and a family's aspirations for their adult child, other families noted that their child was too competent to gain any use out of their centres' basic independence training, as found by another carer:

> They never taught literacy skills! [They thought] 'what would they have done with them? Do something constructive'. She was used to going down the town and they were trying to teach her road-crossing skills. (C17)

In some cases, the extent of person-centred planning in the adaptation of different support options for individuals appeared to be largely in its infancy. A further consequence of the inflexibility in the system is the lack of choice. Carers felt they could either use the local service, even if it was inappropriate, or as an alternative, take nothing. To compound the problem of services being patchy, carers argued that they often could not seek services elsewhere when they were under the umbrella of one service provider. This reflects a lack of consumer choice in disability services.

> If you were going with one service, they won't let you use another. Like at St [Pauls]; he hasn't had speech therapy since August. The speech therapist is on maternity leave. There's only one. And he's not allowed use any other service for speech therapy because he's under the umbrella of St [Pauls]. I mean, they sent me home an information pack to work with him. But I'm not a speech therapist. I do my best but I've two other children. (C3)

Post-School Occupation

As mentioned earlier, the move from adolescence to adulthood is one of the most significant transitions experienced by individuals and their families in terms of finding some type of post-school occupation. At this early stage, many parents were entering into the process of trying to secure some form of work or further training for their son or daughter. Within the broader spectrum of day supports for a young adult with a disability, providing training and support for finding a job was a key aspect of the non-profit disability services' remit.

While the statutory training agency FÁS provides a nationwide Supported Employment Programme (SEP), in reality the non-profit sector support the majority of people with disabilities who require more intensive training. The SEP is a labour market initiative to assist jobseekers with a disability who are 'job ready' to find employment in the open labour market. For the purpose of the Programme, job readiness is defined as 'a person who has the necessary training, education, motivation and ability to pursue work in the open labour market and if needed, has the transport to get to and from work' (FÁS, 2010). In reality then, the non-profit disability service providers have the largest supporting role in helping people to become 'work ready'.

Access to these occupational day services was a crucial issue for many of the families interviewed. Many carers argued that they found it difficult to get a place with the service provider in their designated area. More significantly, many families felt that many of the decisions about the type of services for their adult child were made without their input and were often decided on whether or not there was a 'place' available:

> She wants to do courses, you know, she wants to better herself. So I was just told we have to wait until March to know if there is a place for her. So I said, 'you're actually telling me that you don't know if she's going to be accepted or not?' and now, if she isn't accepted, where do I go from there? (C20)

The fear of leaving school and facing this negotiation of supports is understandable then from this family's experience. As the interviews in the 'Social Workers' section above showed, the lack of information at this crucial time made the accessibility of post-school occupation more difficult.

For many people with less-significant forms of intellectual disability, parents who have high expectations often feel very stressed as they feel that their son or daughter is being held back by the 'disability industry', due to a failure to adopt their services to individual requirements:

> There was no service. I did go to the services when he finished leaving cert. And their attitude had not changed. They still wanted that psychological assessment. They still wanted to put him into a three year training course to figure out what he'd be capable of working at. Which doesn't sound unreasonable. But it didn't take into account his ability at that stage. He went into VITOS [occupational training] and in a week, they had a programme for him. They had no experience of somebody with DS – they devised a programme by simply sitting down and treating him as a normal person. There is an industry around people with disability. And it's not always there to serve the interests of the person who has the disability. Making jobs... (C16)

While person-centred planning has become commonplace within the rhetoric of disability care, these experiences reflect a different reality. The range at which many service providers tailor their supports was quite narrow. There was a general consensus from families about the lack of choice available. If an individual or their family was unhappy with the support options available, generally there was little else available. Most of the carers felt this varied depending on where they lived.

In addition, the quote above also highlights a concern shared by many families, that occupational services still completely underestimated the ability of the person. In certain cases, some providers even recommended sheltered work options. This 'suitability' to sheltered work was often proposed in places where there was no alternative, however. Most carers felt little benefit was gained from working on such community-based employment or training schemes. These schemes rarely led to full-time employment, and the young adult person was caught in a cycle of disability benefits followed by training with little prospect of getting a job in a competitive working environment:

> Yeah.. He was about 18 at the time, They came along and said em.. there's someplace in Naas where he could go and he'd be doing some little job there and they used to pick him up in the morning. But I went in one day to see what he was doing and he was wasting his time – he was rolling strains of wool. I took him out straight away. (C5)

According to *A Strategy for Equality* (1996), employment and training are among the many areas in which people with disabilities are at a disadvantage compared to the rest of society. There are three main consequences of exclusion from the labour market, identified by Berthoud et al. (1993). Firstly, disabled people are being denied the right to work and support themselves. This denies access to the social experience of work and the attached social status. Those who do secure a job are often underemployed in manual, low-skilled occupations and relatively underpaid. Secondly, there are extra living costs for disabled people which have to be met either by the individual or the state. Thirdly, social security payments to support unemployed disabled people are expensive and in many cases are not adequate to maintain the basic, minimum standard of living. Therefore they are more likely to be employed through informal arrangements rather than formal contracts and employment legislation (Murray 1994).

According to the carers interviewed, the experience of trying to find their son or daughter a job in the competitive work environment was difficult and fraught with much anxiety. This often involved the parent making contact themselves with employers and making a request on their child's behalf. Most parents felt that a lot of employers were still fearful of hiring an adult with an intellectual disability, regardless of the level or difficulty of work that would be available. Many carers, such as the example below, spoke of their negative experiences:

> One supermarket owner said to me, 'his staff would feel threatened if he took someone like *that* on'. Now I said to this person, 'how would they feel threatened? Mary is not going to threaten anybody. She's going to go in for a couple of hours a day, if she got the chance, and could stack shelves or tidy up or things like that. What's that threatening?' It's crazy. (C12)

On the other hand, fortunately some carers had positive experiences in getting employment for their adult son or daughter. Although these were generally low-skilled jobs, they offered some degree of job security for the person and the additional benefits outlined above;

> Superquinn and Tesco are good now. Generally after their training-in period, they're able. It is good and it gives them a sense of worth. And it's good for them to be mixing with so-called 'normal' people. (C4)

Although rates of employment for people with disabilities remain low across other countries, including the other two jurisdictions, there are positive approaches being developed such as supported employment. Rather than the traditional ethos to 'train and place', meaning a lengthy training period and then a work placement, supported employment agencies are beginning to realise that a 'place and train' approach is more successful. This means that a person gets their experience *within* a work placement. While this represents a best practice model, in reality, the experiences of families revealed a more haphazard approach is usually taken.

Conclusion

While the last chapter detailed the progression of the broader care system in Ireland for carers in contrast to England and the US, this chapter examined the access to supports accorded to families, and their young adult children at a local scale. As Chapter 3 showed, citizenship is not only conceived as a set of legal obligations and entitlements which individuals possess by virtue of their membership in a state but also the 'right to symbolic presence and visibility (vs. marginalisation); the right to dignifying representation (vs. stigmatisation); and the right to propagation of identity and maintenance of lifestyles (Pakulski, 1997: 80). Throughout this chapter, the carers' narratives demonstrated their strong feelings that the right of recognition was crucial in their ability to access information, education, social services, and respite. Throughout the different sections, it was apparent that there was limited scope for carers to participate in partnership with agencies at the local level, and for agencies to adapt their services to meet the needs of individuals. Moreover, the statutory services often rely on carers within the community care spectrum to carry out the care work alone.

The extent to which the Irish landscape of care works as a system of strategically planned interventions aimed at providing carers with effective support appears, at best, in its infancy. There was a general consensus among carers that the management culture within the statutory and non-profit services was characterised by a lot of 'red tape' and bureaucracy associated with obtaining services. As a result, there was a general reluctance and sense of dread on parents to brave entering into the quagmire of the community care landscape. With the limited role of social workers in guiding families through the process, carers often found accessing appropriate and individualised services to be a lengthy and testing process. This made it difficult for parents to consider and plan for possible changes that could arise with their family's lifestyle, including the financial effects and the restrictions it may impose on their family's social and recreational activities.

On the ground, most of the service needs, in the form of more home-help or respite, were immediate, reflecting the backlog of people awaiting services. The experiences of the carers and carer advocacy groups echoed the figures from the National Intellectual Disability Database (2008), where 242 adults were in need of a day service, with 212 of these with *no* statutory service. From their data, 54.7 per cent of this group had a mild intellectual disability, whose principal requirements included training and employment. The other 39.2 per cent had moderate, severe and profound disability, whose principal requirements were multidisciplinary support services, home support services, special vocational training, and sheltered work (Kelly et al., 2009).

Central to the analysis of these service structures throughout the chapter was an acknowledgement of geographical variations in their delivery. In particular this variation arose from the spatial administration structures of HSEA. The HSEAs played different roles in different areas, in terms of how they arranged their home help services, and in how they designed the contractual relationships with the non-profit sector. At this scale, it is possible to see agency at work, in terms of how proactive a HSEA worked with local agencies. In some cases, the HSEA had their own carer-coordinator to help train and support carers in their local area. While legislation emanates from the state, numerous influences are brought to bear as it is translated and transformed by actors operating at various levels of the policy process – many of which occur within localised contexts. Action by central government is important as it serves as a guideline for interpreting both the spirit and intent of the law. However, unless funding is ring-fenced, and more strategic monitoring is implemented, evidence of strong spatial differences shall no doubt continue to arise. It is therefore only by examining the ways in which policy is mediated by actors operating within and across various spatial and organisational environments, that the connections between care policy and the many local sites within which it is translated and practised can be made.

In a locational sense, it is at the local scale where the tensions between *efficiency* and *effectiveness* essentially create the spatial properties of community care resources (i.e. *where* the *providers* are and why they are there). At this scale, the interviews drew attention to some of the inequities and gaps in spatial distribution between and within health service areas. The ad hoc relationships with the voluntary sector and the bureaucracy involved in service allocation all contributed to disparities between regions. In terms of statutory services, the mixed responses from carers highlighted the makeshift attitude of health professionals towards disability issues. In terms of the statutory/voluntary mix, a major source of regional disparity was the means with which HSEAs fund and allocate tasks to the voluntary organisations. In some areas, there is an obvious commitment to provide community services formally, instead of through the use of voluntary agencies. In other areas, the voluntary sector has, perhaps by necessity, become a much stronger provider of services.

The evidence from the carers and carer groups showed that a top-down approach takes time to penetrate and in many cases dissipated in the middle ground within an administrative jungle. A stronger and more transparent regional counterpart to the government level is lacking. At the delivery level, there is still significant institutional fragmentation. While the bottom-up approach from voluntary organisations is important, a dependence on its organic nature combined with limited monitoring and management has led to considerable gaps in coverage. Care support was therefore not uniform across space and local conditions interact with broader trends to produce specific geographies of care. The evidence from the interviews suggests that the ambiguous nature of family care between formal/informal, public/private responsibilities is still evident in social policy. This means that social rights, in contrast to civil and political rights, are indeed largely viewed as political programmes. In this way, Drewett's (1999) assertion that social rights are not 'rights' at all, but instead are akin to party manifestos, appears largely accurate for family carers.

Chapter 8
Socio-spatial Experiences of Carers

As discussed in the last chapter, the implications of living in a service system discussed in the last chapter has significant effects on family carers. This chapter looks at the physical, emotional and psychological effects on carers, highlighting the social and spatial experiences of being in such a landscape of care. Concepts of space and place are shown to be helpful in understanding issues and experiences of caregiving. As Wiles (2003) argues, the social and the physical aspects of the many interconnected scales and places which caregivers negotiate on an everyday basis both shape and are shaped by caregiving.

Wiles (2003) examines three spatial scales at which caregiving is experienced; the body, the household, and beyond. At each scale, the emphasis is on the inter-related and connected nature of the social and physical aspects of caregiving. The quantity and nature of the work relating to the body has an enormous impact on the daily life of the caregiver and their household. As well as the physical impacts of caregiving, the carer also has to care for a body imbued with many social meanings – such as the negative attitudes towards disability. While these experiences are largely social and emotional, they have consequences on the carers' daily geographies, such as limiting their home range and negatively affecting their everyday social interactions and ability to work. The experiences of carers as explored in this chapter resonate with Wiles' explication of the three interconnected scales; moreover, it is possible to discern from their narratives the significant effect of living within a broader landscape of care provision at each of these scales.

The Intangible Caregiving Relationship

Grappling with Independence

Becoming a carer often means having to learn about topics and issues that one would never have had to deal with before, some of which may not be immediately obvious. Caregiving shapes multiple aspects of a carer's life, including their daily geographies and everyday experiences. This forces a renegotiation of home, public spaces, mobility, family and identity (Dyck, 1995, 1998). As the following sections demonstrate, carers of young adults with intellectual disabilities both share similar experiences in common with wider caregiving experiences and at the same time, have unique and particular experiences different from caring for people with physical disability, or frail elderly persons.

Generally the families spoke of having fewer physical tasks than those looking after someone with a physical disability. Exceptions to this occurred for a number of carers who had to carry out routine physical or 'medical' tasks for the care recipient due to more severe or multiple disabilities. However, for the majority, the tasks involved were inherently non-technical. Most families felt that it is the long hours minding and *promoting the independence* of the person which caused exhaustion and the limitations on their freedom. Such care is not an area where one social support institution can claim unique competency in its provision. As a result there is no natural division of labour among family caregivers, home-helps recruited from the market place, and state subsidised providers in meeting the non-medical needs of the care recipient (Soldo and Freedman, 1994).

In terms of *promoting the independence* of the person, this was perhaps the most difficult and time-consuming part of the work of a caregiver. Many of the carers talked about being regularly exhausted due to the extra rigour of keeping the person stimulated and occupied. This intimate task features largely in the qualitative experience of caring throughout the study. Again, this is a very different experience for carers of persons for intellectual disability as opposed to other forms of disability, in that someone with a physical disability can motivate themselves to overcome their barriers. More often, as the following two quotes show, the parent with an intellectually disabled son or daughter has to play the role of advocate and provide the motivation:

> You want the person with the disability to be independent. You don't want them to be institutionalised [after you're gone]. He's not that independent, I *make* him go places. We'd say we're going to the football match, 'c'mon get your coat!'. Whereas you could sit at home and do nothing. (C13, original emphasis)

> Just being around where he is. I mean I make the dinner anyway, that's no big deal anyway. But it's more the fact that you need to be around. Not the fact that you have to do a huge amount of things for him. You'd plan things for him if you're going out. You'd be saying to him, 'well we're going into town, you'll need your jacket'. You know, things like that. Making sure he's taking his tablets. I don't have to do things for him. He needs guidance. (C3)

These quotes demonstrate a more nuanced picture of the subtle tasks that many families engage in. They are elusive to definition, yet require much time and dedication. As a result, carers in general felt that they needed a great degree of patience to communicate and explain phenomena that go on in everyday life. Sometimes, there is a slower adaptive learning curve on the part of the disabled adult, and changes in the pattern of the daily routine can sometimes cause confusion. While the learning curve can be slower and the person can have a different mode of thinking, depending on the type of learning difficulty, generally an adult can be facilitated to achieve a degree of independence. This often can only be achieved though if the different mode of thinking is facilitated in family life:

> It just doesn't suit the program. It must fit his program. And he can't just catch things sometimes now. Like he can't, no matter what the situation, admit it's not his fault. If he's in trouble, it's not his fault, it's your fault. 'I couldn't be wrong'. It's tough. He's all go all the time. It must fit his program. And he can't just catch things sometimes now. He just does his own thing. [Carescapes] could get him to do things but for us to get him to do anything else. You cannot order him around. But I think, if you get around him in a nice way. (C22)

Because of the large time investment required in facilitating and advocating the development of the disabled person, it therefore requires a distinct duty of care. In most cases, the duty of care was evident in the narratives of the carer. In particular, this was most evident in relation to promoting the independence of their adult child, and planning on the development for their future. In the following two excerpts, it is possible to discern the sense of responsibility that parents took in relation to this:

> Once [Michael] came along, it just wasn't possible [to return to work] because of the path we chose with him. I was the one providing all the information to the school, helping with the homework every day. It was a big commitment, even researching how to teach, but it meant a commitment every single day and it meant being there every day. It was time consuming, but it was also very draining emotionally because people would always say to you, 'ah he's grand now, but what are you going to do when he's 7 or 8, he might get into the primary school but what happens when he gets there'? And then when he got through primary school, 'you don't think he's going to go through exams, do you?' [Laughs]. But it wasn't about exams really. It was about being part of the community. It was about knowing people in the community. I mean, his whole social life is around the people he grew up with. So that's what stopped me from working. (C9)

In the quote, the carer's assertion that being part of the community was so important for her son was telling. One of the most significant challenges facing adults with intellectual disabilities, many carers felt, was isolation and loneliness. Being at school in the earlier years helped in knowing people in the community. Maintaining a social life into adulthood around those that the person grew up with often becomes a significant focus of the caregiver. In addition, families often had to create 'intentional communities'.

Whether all carers invest this time appeared to be largely dependent on their individual sense of duty. As one of the carers put it, she feels obliged to provide full-time care, but acknowledges her failure at meeting the requirements of this task. In the following two excerpts, it is possible to see the weight of obligation in their lives:

> I have been very involved over the years. I still do as much as I can. I'm not on the committee, I'd prefer not to. I do what I can, I'll help fundraise and I'll watch everything which goes on. My heart is willing, but the flesh is weak. I want to do so much. Having someone with special needs can have a good effect on a family. But then if you had a wish in the morning... you could wish it away too. It can be a minefield. No two situations are the same. I hear some hair-raising stories. There's a lovely family in [Kildare] where the mother has breakdown after breakdown. (C17)

> It's a thing you just do, when it comes to the family, you just do it. I heard someone say to me recently, 'I couldn't do it'. Well I said, what if it was for your mother or your husband? If you were dropped in the deep end, you'd just have to do it. (C1)

These family carer experiences illustrate that the extent their sense of duty was shaped by social norms feeding into expectations of parental practices. With the exception of one carer who willingly accepted that she was seeking a residential 'group home' placement for her son, in general, the sense of duty was shared by most.

In terms of grappling with independence, the wider support services appeared to play a crucial role in shaping carer judgements. Some looking after adults with less-severe forms of intellectual disability had to confront the negative assumptions about the disability themselves. The effect of a physician's early broad diagnosis and school staff not recognising the ability of the person made it difficult for the carer to challenge these broad assumptions later. It is only with experience, that the carer can ascertain the specific ability of the person. However, as the following quote reveals, the level of expectation differed greatly between families in what their child could achieve, thus demonstrating the degree of agency in caregiver's lives. Investing the time in the non-technical supportive functions of caregiving was very much a personal attribute; some had fundamental feelings of wanting more for their child than currently available from the services:

> Really, the diagnosis of DS doesn't predict development. But if you are constantly told he'll never do this, or he'll never do that, then it really does colour your judgement. I suppose I'm the kind of person who if you tell me I can't do something, I try it. Now some professionals would say, you're denying reality, if you talk like that. Do you know? Again, I suppose it's what you want for your child. There are parents who are quite happy to have their son or daughter go to a service where they go bowling on Monday, they go swimming on Tuesday, they go to football on Wednesday. But that's not what I want for Michael because I don't think we would be doing him any service…allowing him to have a life of pleasure. Like I mean, we'd all like a life of pleasure but it would get very boring

> after a couple of weeks. And I think mentally, he wouldn't benefit in the long run. There would be a deterioration. (C16)

While motivation and stimulus, as indicated above, in promoting independence was a seminal theme in the parents' narratives, at the same time, many of the carers' were fraught with fears over the protection of their child. Overprotection on the part of carers is seldom addressed in the literature, and is a key issue for parents and the development of the child. Despite the efforts to promote independence, throughout the study, it was not uncommon for parents of young adults with intellectual disabilities to be ill-prepared in dealing with issues around encouraging independence when there was perceived risk involved. While most just want their disabled son or daughter to be able to look after themselves, at the same time, some found it quite shocking for them to exhibit much more independence that they thought possible. For children without disabilities, it is usual for parents to learn to facilitate their child's emerging needs and desires as they develop. However, the presence of a learning difficulty can compound this parenting skill. Therefore, in many cases, parents make all decisions, instead of trying to facilitate the choices of the disabled person. In one instance, a family carer was able to admit being over-protective herself:

> Do you think some parents are over-protective? Oh yeah I could fall into that category very easily myself. I would really. I try not to. Oh Jee, am I aware of it? [Laughs]. I suppose with [Sarah], inside our hearts we are. (C17)

The same carer told a story of her reaction to her child, after she decided to travel home herself without any forward planning:

> She had her bags one day and missed the bus home from town. No word from her. She hadn't rang. I was beginning to panic. She pulled into the taxi rank and got a lift home. She said 'Mam, don't make a fuss'.
>
> *Are you fearful about that?*
>
> My own fears? We're very attached. Dangerously attached. She worries about me. It's ok of course but I don't know how you detach it. That's a silly question. I really don't know how to separate us. She's just a magnet in the house…going 24. (C17)

This close-bond is evident in many other caregiving relationships where fears about risk are evident. In another instance of this struggle with granting choice and freedom, it is clear to see the close-bonds between a carer and her adult daughter. In the following quote, a family carer and her adult daughter appear to be very close, and the parent's anxiety about allowing her daughter walk around town is reflected in her happy willingness to assist her:

> She's not all that bad. I mean she can walk from here down to the bookshop. The only thing is I don't like her crossing where the lights are down the town. But that's all. But since I retired, I could go down with her. She's clever enough with money and that. We look after her benefit, we pay it into the credit union for her. She's very hard to get money out of. [Laughs] (C20)

Rather than according blame on parents for restricting the life-choices of young people with disabilities which often appears in the literature (see Twigg and Atkin, 1994), the narratives of the families revealed a more nuanced account of this caregiving relationship. One of the main reasons for carers' feelings of overprotection appeared to be the lack of counselling and social work that could encourage parents to gauge what degree of freedom would be appropriate for their sons or daughters to attain. A strong paternal ethos often still resides in services, given the liability of risks, and their health and safety protocols. These appear to also have an effect on families:

> What happens with the family then, is they become nearly more protective. Because if a service provider is saying, 'oh god, we couldn't mind him, he'd need three people', then they're not even going to ask their relatives to take him for a weekend. Because they're saying well if they can't, our sister surely can'*t. So it does colour the whole thinking on the situation.* A lot of the time, the people you see walking up the town, taking someone with Down's Syndrome by the hand; it's almost accentuating their disability. I think they're a very empathic people – people with DS you know, they really live up or down to your expectations. And if you believe that he or she would never be capable of something, then a lot of the time, that's what happens. I think that's the saddest thing for people starting off. Nowadays – their dreams are taken away. There's no reason nowadays why somebody with DS can't have a very fulfilled independent life. As a parent, you have to [check] yourself a lot of the time and say 'ok, I have to let go'. And letting go is difficult. But that isn't something that the service providers instil in families. (C16)

In addition to the role of professionals, feelings of over-protection appeared to also arise from social norms – which assume the dependency of a disabled person – feeding into expectations of parental practices. For one older carer, who had cared for her disabled adult son for 40 years, admitted resisting against these social norms. In this instance, she comments on younger parents today being more protective in comparison with her own generation:

> He was late walking and one time, this woman said to me 'is that child not walking yet?' I said, 'no, he crawls', so she said, 'you know what to do with him: Get a tea chest and put him in the tea chest, and you wait till you see, he'll be walking. Because he'll want to stand up and see what's going on'. And she was perfectly right. With all the so-called psychology, they would probably say

> you were cruel. Like some people say, 'playpens are bad'. Well my God, I had my two grandchildren in playpens, and their mother would say that [playpens] were awful. So it's gone to the other extreme […]. I met a woman who was going to town by bus and she had a Down's Syndrome with her and I told her Paddy went with the darts team and she said she just didn't let him. Too much protection!…and maybe she lived on her own. (C5)

Coping with the Particular Emotional Aspects

The intangible caregiving tasks outlined in the previous section, such as motivating, promoting independence, and dealing with overprotection, had clear implications for each of the family members involved. As well as the huge time investment in these tasks, caring for another person can potentially lead to considerable physical exhaustion and emotional distress for both. As this section outlines, the narratives from the carers demonstrate that the emotional aspect of care work, particularly for a young adult with intellectual disabilities is just as important, if not more so, than the physical tasks.

Firstly, many of the carers talked about being regularly exhausted due to the extra rigour of keeping the person stimulated and occupied in order to encourage their independence. With this level of dedication, it was not surprising that most carers talked about being physically tired by the long days involved in meeting this commitment at home, as well as additional commitments many carers had, such as participating in local support and advocacy groups. Consequently, many speak of being at tired and frustrated with the long days involved:

> When it comes to 10 o'clock at night, I just feel I've had enough with it. It's every day. And [Sarah] is 18 years old now, and from the time she was born, I've travelled up and down the country on public transport to hospitals for her. I've left home at maybe half nine in the morning and won't get home till 6 o'clock because I'm on public transport. She would get very angry, and say "well why did you have me?" So there's a lot of anger. It's understandable. They say the one closest to you, is the one that can give you most heartbreak. (C3)

In terms of the emotional effects, because of the close nature of the caregiving relationship, carers can sometimes get upset, when their child gets frustrated. The mood or behaviour of the care recipient can have direct implications on the way the carer felt. This means that, at times, carers can experience emotional stress caused by a negative frame of mind from the care recipient:

> There are times when I get upset and I keep saying "these people are just upset" and just try and put it in perspective without recognising that I might be upset about the fact that names are being called at me (C25).

From these moments a carer can sometimes feel that their work goes unrecognised and unappreciated. A carer's emotional responses and coping strategies were particularly challenged when their adult son or daughter appeared unappreciative of their efforts, and duty of care weighs heavily on them:

> Yeah sometimes I'm not allowed to say that I'm tired, or I'm fed-up, or I'm upset, or I'm going through a bad patch because I don't think they realise that everyone has to carry their own cross (C25).

The emotional nature of this type of care work was regarded as more important by most of the carers therefore, than any physical tasks. This was similar to Wiles (2003) findings for carers of frail, elderly people.

Some carers were acutely aware that institutional accommodation may be the only option available to their sibling after the carer passes away. Worrying about the care needs of the recipient in the long-term was a key feature of the caregiving experience. Therefore trying to find whether or not other family members will take over the reins is an important consideration which carers like to resolve:

> I know nobody should worry about the future but you do. You want the person with the disability to be independent or whether your other children will take him on. That is a problem. You don't want them to be institutionalised. (C12)

> The only fear we have is after we pass on – if she can be looked after as good as we looked after her. No one can say she will. I mean people will promise the sun, moon and stars and you can't plan for it. But we're hoping she will be looked after. (C20)

Trying to remain optimistic is the most common coping strategy expressed by carers, yet this leaves many potential problems unresolved. However, being optimistic was essential for their peace of mind, and many tried to remain hopeful that changes would happen in the community care system, which would advance the chances of the individual to remain independent in their community:

> Yeah. I have to be optimistic. Or else I can't go on. It needs legislation that people will have rights based education and the right to get employment like everybody else. The right to live wherever they want to live. (C12)

Some families had actively planned for the future as a way of addressing these issues and for giving peace of mind. One family ensured that the house was put in the name of the person they were looking after. On the other hand, while everyone had thought about the future, some carers could not face dealing with it and had not yet put plans in place for the care of the person:

> *Do you worry about the future?*
>
> Well that's the main thing of course. You can't think about it too much. That's my attitude. I know that might be dodging the issue, but you don't want it hanging over your head. (C13)

Often their fear of changing circumstances arise from the carer's direct relationship with the state. Many felt that because of their dependence on state support, they were susceptible to fluctuations in resources and staffing within the community care services:

> We're going to lose that girl now at Christmas – she's going to have a baby. So I'm looking for someone else at the moment. I mean the stress levels are terrible. (C3)

As a result, many of the emotions tied up with caregiving, in particular their anxiety about the future, are largely a result of their vulnerability and exposure to changing circumstances of the 'outside' landscape of care.

This is aggravated by the economic position of the family. Normally, a family's economic position can be expected to fluctuate throughout its lifecycle. It starts when its children are young, eases as the children grow up and leave home or contribute financially to the household, and returns as the stage of retirement is reached (Cecil et al., 1987: 62). However, where a family is dependent on state benefits or a low income, the presence of a family member with a disability can lead to additional challenges. Most family carers make significant economic sacrifices by quitting their jobs, working part-time, or not seeking employment at all. There is also a loss of income from earnings when a carer is forced to reduce hours of work or forego promotion opportunities because of the commitments of the caring role. In addition, carers often require a variety of commodities that help to make life easier, including practical assistance for the disabled person. All of these pressures affect carers which means that they – or their adult child – often face an uncertain future. Therefore anxiety about the long-term future features highly in carers' minds. According to one carer: *"The sad fact is that most people find time to rest in life, while carers cannot even rest in peace"* (C25). Carers of disabled adults are concerned about who will care for their children when they die, or how they will be able to finance formal care if they become too old and frail to cope.

Unfortunately for carers who have no other children, the choices of somebody to take over the caring duties are more limited. In any case, most of the carers were anxious to lay all the responsibility of caring on the other family members. The needs of spouses and children were also considered and negotiated. For some families, relying on others within the family to take over the role of caring was too much to expect, and was regarded as especially hard for their other sons or daughters. In the following quote, a family carer who has two daughters with intellectual disabilities expressed her fears:

> *In terms of the future, do you worry about it?*
>
> I do, yeah. My own children have said, look don't worry, we'll look after them. My second son said he will stand for [Amy], but he's married now and has 2 children so I don't know what is going to happen. My older daughter is very good but I'm just worried if something happened to me in the morning. Where's it all going to end? I mean, I was knocked down in October. Two cars crashed and went up on the footpath. I was in hospital and I don't think there was anywhere I could have called to ask could they take the girls? (C14)

Caring for adults with an intellectual disability is perhaps unique in this respect, in that helping them develop general independence skills can have the most significant positive effects in alleviating the carers' stress of worrying about their future. The earlier development of the care recipient's independent living skills is therefore crucial and usually has positive repercussions in other areas of their lives. The establishment of an adequate social life should also have positive effects in helping develop general independence skills and establishing a more active and integrated role in the community. This is a worthwhile investment for family carers as it enables the young person to gain competence at living more independently later (Redmond, 1996: 31).

Throughout the interviews there were positive signs that this was the case. Despite the high levels of stress and physical and mental exhaustion admitted by the participants, they did agree strongly however on the positive emotional aspects of caring in terms of how it has positively changed their own personal attitudes.

The personal rewards were evident from the carers, such as seeing the disabled adult progress. Being able to acknowledge the positive aspects of having a child with a disability appeared to be a feature particular to carers of an *adult* with intellectual disabilities, as opposed to a child, given the length of time the relationship between the two has developed. In addition to understanding disability better, the carers felt that they had a better understanding for people in any situation. According to one carer: *"You have a more open mind with any problems other people have, anything at all"* (C24). Being in an environment which is marginalised in many ways from the general public had implications on the way carers felt about able-bodied people: *"People really do get wrapped up in their own world, running around and something suddenly happens"* (C25). A general consensus among the participants therefore was that because of their caregiving role, they felt that they could more easily put things into perspective.

These intangible aspects of caregiving, in particular from caring for young adults with intellectual disabilities – grappling with independence and coping with the particular emotional aspects – have potentially strong geographical effects. Moreover, different spaces can markedly shape these aspects of everyday caregiving. The remainder of this chapter explores how these aspects play out across scale, from the public sphere to the private home sphere and in-between. It becomes clear that the intangible aspects become more 'real' in everyday lived space; as the carer must negotiate different codes of practice and expectations in different places.

Public Encounters – Caring for a 'Disabled' Person

In caring for someone with an intellectual disability, it is not only the cognitive impairment that shapes the carer's experiences. More specifically, a carer has to deal with outside social responses, public policies and public attitudes. Carers are confronted with dealing with the *representation* of the disabled body in society and the experiences of embodiment. This is compounded by the proximity of the care recipient to the carer throughout life. Proximity is a key theme of geographic research on informal caregiving. Proximity affects the likelihood, nature and intensity of providing care (Wiles, 2003). Difficulties can arise in the relationship between the carer and the care recipient due to the close proximity of co-existence. Even where much affection exists between a carer and their young adult son or daughter, there may be occasional or frequent difficulties in the relationship (Cecil et al., 1987: 66). Sibley suggests that close proximity heightens the urge to expel; 'spatial proximity weakens the social distance between self and other and challenges the integration of individual identity' (1995: 11). At the scale of the body, there is a risk that the lives of people in a caring relationship might become so inextricably entwined that one individual can have no independence of the other; particularly outside the home. Many carers talked about travelling everywhere with their son or daughter, whether they go shopping, to the library, or to visit other households. The main reason for this was that busy public places or some day care programmes appeared to have negative effects on the mentality and temperament of some adults with intellectual disabilities:

> Oh yeah there has to be someone around – we used to rely a lot on day care but [James] used to get scared and went in to himself a lot so then we used to take turns. We then had to try and draw him out again. (C3)

Because carers felt concern for the safety of their care recipient, breaks tended to be shorter and were characterised by 'popping down to the shops' or 'going for a coffee in town'. Even those who could leave the person alone often talked about how they would have a bad conscience if anything should happen.

While carers' and their adult child's geographies extended beyond the home, the issue of being comfortable with the disabled person in public space was a dominant theme addressed by carers. This was particularly an issue that carers grappled with in 'the earlier days' when the carers' son or daughter was younger:

> I'll never forget when she was a baby, we were in town that day, and I met a friend. And she just ignored the fact that I had a baby... just because she was Down's. I was distraught. I was shattered. (C17)

While this carer had since developed more resilient coping strategies, as discussed later, it nonetheless demonstrates the immediate impact that carers are confronted with in negotiating public 'meetings' in everyday life. Another carer argued that in public space, while people did not actively discriminate against people with disabilities, nevertheless they generally did not understand disability: *"All I notice is ignorance...ignorance in the kinder sense of the word"* (C18). Similarly, another carer argued that society has a long way to come to accept disability: *"society hasn't opened up much to people with disabilities – to a certain degree they have, but no... they have a long way to go"* (C24). This largely stems from the general public's fear or reluctance to engage with certain people with intellectual disabilities; particularly if they demonstrate different behaviour. Some carers mentioned that often people ask them a question about their son or daughter, despite being in the latter's company. These interactions are often due to the awkwardness felt by an able-bodied person during personal encounters; *"I sometimes get that, where people talk to me about more serious things than they would with [Mark]"* (C5). These moments can sometimes cause discomfort for the son or daughter, and thus can make the carer feel momentarily awkward.

Often carers spoke of everyday interactions being more difficult in busy places, where people had less time to be patient:

> We're becoming a lot harsher, especially in Dublin. I notice when I go into a shop or something…there isn't as much tolerance anymore…with fumbling with their change, or if somebody can't manage something. (C25)

It was also highlighted that carers and their adult children have similar expectations and standards about places as able-bodied people do. This may not be immediately obvious to the general public or their attempt at addressing the issue of access. As voiced by one carer: *"I mean just cause some place is accessible, the food could be terrible and it might not suit"* (C1). Therefore the fact that a specific site may be accessible does not directly mean that someone with a disability chooses to include it in their daily maps of use; often the attitudinal reactions from staff played a more important role.

While these sentiments expressed the level of disappointment at the way the general public were often ignorant or awkward with people with disabilities, carers also felt they had to *confront* or *divert* society's discomfort and behaviour face-to-face. This was another outcome of proximity, as evidenced throughout the interviews, where there was a knock-on effect of negative perceptions of disability by the general public on the carer. In describing many awkward instances with able-bodied people, carers regularly had to face people in hybrid states of awkwardness, confusion, and distraction. Referring to the words of Thomson (1997), in talking about an encounter with a person with a visible disability, 'it almost always dominates and skews the normate's (sic) process of sorting out perceptions and forming a reaction' (p. 12). In other words, often the young adult and their carer have to 'meet' people in heightened senses of discomfort. As a result, carers generally felt they had complex geographies of public life, managing people's reactions. This was illustrated by the experiences of one of the carers:

> Well you'd come across a few barriers now with a child like [Deirdre] that has Down's Syndrome. They're kinda very uneasy. They don't expect her to be as normal as she is. Do you know, they look at her, they know she's Downs, but they kinda treat her like a child, even though she's an adult. And she doesn't like that at all. She likes her drop of Bailey's. And people are shocked then. (C4)

Although the hybrid state of the person is generally transient, the fact that carers have to face these again and again makes it difficult for them to deal with the public in a way they perhaps would have, without the person with the disability. Therefore their everyday geographies are often skewed by such experience. Carers mentioned that they were always aware of codes of behaviour or attitudes regarding expected social norms in particular places, hence calling into question their ability to presume their able-bodiedness, as others may unconsciously do. Re-thinking their own embodied space called into question their own place-in-the-world. At the root of these concerns was an awareness of the way in which their son or daughter may react in public interactions: *"You can't go to mass because you don't know how he's going to react...so you're very limited"* (C25). Throughout the interviews, the participants recounted many awkward moments that took place in public, which tended to arise from interactions with people. Similar experiences were expressed by the following two parents:

> You have to be aware of people's needs as well, what they want. (C3)

> You have to be sensitive to everybody's needs...You have to be fairly tuned in all around. (C25)

These sentiments highlight the way many of the participants felt in shared public space. Being in a more public environment can expose the carer to competing and sometimes-conflicting understandings of, and comments about, what is 'good' caregiving (Wiles, 2003). In response to this, some of the carers felt that they often had to make the extra effort to make people feel comfortable in interactions with the person with the disability.

Fortunately, over time most carers had developed various coping strategies to feel more comfortable taking their adult son or daughter out in public. Most carers talked about a certain level of discomfort, but most of the time, this did not affect their mobility *with* the person anymore:

> I used to feel uncomfortable when I found children staring at her. I got annoyed at that, but sure they were only children – they don't know any better. I feel definitely that much more should be expected from people. Say you're out in a restaurant. I find if he misbehaves, people kind of stare at you. He's got to be

> socially acceptable in his behaviour. He can't be carrying on or anything, as a normal child would get away with. (C7)

Most had a well-organised routine in dealing with public responses to the disability. This shows how caregivers are not passive 'victims' of a role, but are quite active in formulating and exercising coping strategies (Wiles, 2003). Many would state the fact that their child had a disability, thus deflecting the onus back onto a member of the public who was staring or looking uncomfortable:

> People would be looking at him. Because he looks normal. I don't care anymore. It's funny their reaction when you say he's special needs. They back off. I'm always a great believer in telling people if he's screaming or shouting. The doctor told me, 'if you're under stress and he's carrying on, just turn around and say, he's special needs'. It takes it all off you. Then it's on them on how to react. (C3)

Practical coping strategies like this were highlighted in many of the carer's interviews. While this resolved many awkward moments, at the same time, it unfortunately perpetuated negative notions of disability, as it naturalised certain forms of behaviour as 'being disabled'

Carers had also developed routines that would regulate access to public space. Some had very straightforward consistent guidelines, or places which were 'out-of-bounds' as regards their everyday life, such as one carer who argued;

> We have to lock all the doors. Or else bring him everywhere. I suppose I've got used to it now. I mean, he couldn't go out there and play out there with the other children. Oh, he'd just keep going. Or else he'd go with anyone. He trusts everybody. (C3)

According to Wiles (2003), routines help to ensure the comfort of recipients through structure, help caregivers manage the demands of their day, and help mitigate the stress of crises. Depending on the severity of the disability, recreational trips can be difficult with considerable work involved in getting ready. Outings of all kinds can involve a great deal of organisation and preparation. The participants mentioned that they had to restructure their own routines in many ways. One of the carers argued that instead of being able to head off somewhere, she had to organise and maintain a routine, only being allowed to go somewhere when organised in advance:

> Yes you'd have to have a routine. Everything has to be planned and then sometimes you can't go. It might depend on the way [Orla] is. I mean, your lifestyle changes. If you want to go away, you have to do way more planning with regard to getting away. (C21)

As the previous two quotes demonstrated, in terms of leaving the home space, often carers felt they were reluctant to let their son or daughter go out on their own. While this varied from parent to parent, and from disability to disability, it shows the decisions parents have to go through to confront their own fears as well as having to grapple with societies' expectations and risks. Many reported that when they needed to go outside the home, they had to bring the person and continue to care. Thus even outside the home, many carers still did not have freedom from the routines of caregiving.

In terms of getting a better sense of carers' perceptions of broader society, many felt the charity mentality was still very evident from the general public: *"there is this charity element about it. You know, we are the able-bodied, and they are disabled, they are disadvantaged"* (C5). This often negates the sense of people with disabilities being active citizens themselves. This charity mentality, according to many families therefore sets up a structure of inequality that reduces the status of their child with disabilities:

> Oh yeah, majorly. This pity, 'oh God bless the poor soul'. We went to a basketball ground and we got lost. And Sheenah, said, 'Jesus Christ where is the basketball ground?', and the looks we got off people! I said Sheenah, we need to go back to the car. It was the same with the Special Olympics. I couldn't get into all that hype. I feel like saying, 'lady, we have the Special Olympics here all the time. It didn't take New Zealand to come to Naas surely, to make you aware'. They exist here too. I found myself really angry. (C17)

The hosting of the Special Olympics in Ireland, as referenced by this carer, saw a major increase in the visibility in people with disabilities in public life. Most carers thought it had a positive effect on people's attitudes, yet were cautious to envisage a longer-term change.

It was also mentioned that people's behaviour can often completely change when they realise that the person they are dealing with has a disability, thus causing embarrassment and awkwardness. One carer talked about an incident in a supermarket, where the store manager started giving out to their adult child because he was shouting, however as soon as he realised he was disabled, he became embarrassed and began apologising. Many others echoed these sentiments. This can even be the case with extended family members:

> It's strange now though. My Mother, she couldn't accept [Paddy], not really. Because I would sometimes say to her "[Paddy] did this, [Paddy] did that, isn't it marvellous?" She never reacted. You know? I was surprised with my mother because she was quite modern in her outlook. But maybe that is just too much for some people to accept. But I always console myself that so called "sane" people are to me often bloody insane and stupid. (C5)

Another serious point mentioned was that very few people get to know disabled people. This critical assertion highlights one of the largest barriers which people with disabilities must face. The fact that people do not get to know or understand them, means that their fear of disabled people is maintained. One family who owned a pub stated:

> I would say now, being here in the pub they would be more aware of things because of [Mary]. Because they all know of [Mary]. So they would be more alert in their own way about it. But the general public doesn't bother. They don't. They're not being educated. (C19)

As a result, families still found it was hard for their disabled son or daughter to make personal friends. Carers felt that people were losing out because of physical and attitudinal barriers. According to Dear et al. (1997), the production of difference is characterised as necessarily a social and a spatial process, which allows the self to be partitioned from the other:

> A lot of people would kind of crouch away from her. And even little kids would stare. You don't mind little children but adults should understand it a little bit better. But I suppose that all goes back to years ago where they were put into institutions when they were babies. It is amazing that people are still clueless... (C25)

Thus it was found that carers share a similar understanding of their surroundings as the care recipient, as a result of the social construction of their identity, and that of someone with a disability. This was evidenced in the similarities in the way carers perceived the care recipient's attitudinal barriers. As a result, some carers felt that, they had a *dual-identity* where their 'carer' identity was separate to their 'personal' identity. Moreover, many felt that 'being a carer' did not fit their personal character. Because of the negative attitudes towards disability and the notion of 'difficult' parents from the health services, this led some to dislike the admission of being a carer:

> I hated this admission; "my child is handicapped". It's the admission. It was saying, "oh do I have to do this?" We were lucky. [Gill] was healthy. But for some reason, when she was 16, I just didn't want to tell the world my child is officially handicapped…I didn't want that. It is like an identity being forced upon you. That's exactly it. I was avoiding it. I just didn't want it. Whether you like it or not, you're forced into this relationship with health and social services. (C17)

This emotional and social coping strategy resonates with recent geographical work on embodiment, emphasising the interconnectedness of the emotional and physical nature of bodies (Parr, 2002).

While it was clear that the carers interviewed all experienced the same exclusionary attitudes and problems, most had different ways of coping, due to different philosophies, attitudes, personalities, and gender role expectations. The complexity and contradictory nature of the relationship between carer and care recipient meant each caregiving scenario was different, with mixed feelings of love, anger, frustration, guilt and concern. According to one carer:

> From the point of view of how well we coped, there was another child born with Down's Syndrome at the same time as [Nicola]. Now if you were to talk to [Ms Tracy], her experience was completely the opposite to ours. Yet it started exactly the same time. So you might say, you have to grieve the child that you expect, and accept the child you have. But you will find that if you put two people on the same road, and the same thing happens to them, yet their observations of the experiences are completely the opposite. (C21)

Therefore how people interpret a situation has a bearing on their experience of caregiving (Luk, 2002). While some actively resist and challenge the troubles facing them through direct protest, many others exhibit forms of self-regulation. For instance, caregivers may frame things as everyday or normal, or alternatively emphasise their ability to handle a crisis situation unconsciously forming a coping strategy. Many others feel concern and guilt over feeling angry thus exhibiting a form of self-regulation. The social and spatial effects of caregiving is reproduced with little challenge, and is made out to be common-sense, as reflected by Bourdieu's (1991) notion of doxa, an unconscious acceptance, or the taken-for-granted, way of things.

As a result of the physical, emotional and psychological impacts on carers identified in this section, particularly in public space, mobility was a key theme that emerged in the lives of carers. In the case of family carers of young adults with intellectual disabilities, their mobility appeared to be shaped as much by the social and emotional factors as the physical ones. As part of their everyday life, carers often had to face attitudinal barriers, as a result of negative feelings or ignorance towards people with disabilities. By the nature of their work, carers are indirectly affected by such attitudinal barriers. Due to the carers' concern and sense of duty for the safety of the care recipient, their daily space and focus of their energy is restricted to the needs of the recipient, and often confined to the household. As a result, their mobility was considerably restricted.

Tied to the Home

Some carers, as touched on in the previous section, were very conscious of the narrowness of their lives, while others appeared to have adapted or resigned themselves to it. The need of some disabled people for constant care and attention can result in a carer being *tied to the home*. One of the most fundamental concerns addressed by carers therefore appeared to be the limits on their home range. Many of the family carers admitted that the constraints on their freedom was the worst thing they had to deal with. There are also profound knock-on effects which are expressed in areas of social and family life. Generally there is a strong tendency to contain problems within the household; often members of the family who live outside the household are assumed to be busy with their own immediate family and are not expected to contribute very much. The twin difficulties of finding people who express a willingness to 'mind' their disabled son or daughter and the reticence of many carers to ask, means that sometimes, carers may rarely go out on normal family outings. This could be a further factor contributing to the reported deterioration in the carer's everyday geographical lifeworld:

> I still am very tied to the home. Because I can't have a job. I could never have had a job after [Cliona]. I wouldn't like to leave her too long. She's never been away on her own, without me. So she's at home with mam, all the rest of the time. And nobody else added. (C19)

Another part of the reason the carers felt tied to the home was that the person being cared for did not like to go away for larger stretches of time. The home space and the routine associated with being around the home offered a degree of safety and security. This made it very difficult for the family sometimes to go away on holiday:

> She doesn't like travelling, she doesn't like being away from her home environment. She'd sooner be in [our neighbours] than with her brothers. But she won't come away with us. Even around Ireland. She likes to come in and out.
>
> *Would you feel tied to the home?*
>
> Yeah. Yeah. But I mean we're quite happy to look after her. (C20)

However, while the home offered a secure, somewhat therapeutic environment, many carers talked about their adult child's reluctance to be *left alone* within the house, thus exacerbating the restraints on carers' mobility. A significant effect on their mobility therefore was their lack of freedom to leave the house *without* the person they're caring for. In other words, getting away from the home, without having to bring the person was a crucial geographical constraint.

> I can leave the house for an hour or so. But he doesn't really like it; being left alone. He wouldn't touch anybody, he'd probably be ok but I suppose I'd be a bit apprehensive. But normally I take him everywhere with me. (C4)

One of the most direct implications of the mobility restrictions identified, as well as of a carer's perceived metaphorical 'place' in society, as argued by the carers, appeared to be the limits on their home range. Geographically, this led to a shifting and dynamic relationship between typically 'private' and 'public' space and parts of the home. In some cases, there was an actual physical change to the homespace. Some carers had to make structural changes to their home, due to some adults having additional impairments or medical needs. In these cases, the house itself had to be renovated to accommodate for wheelchairs, and other equipment.

More often though it was the *meaning* of the homespace that changed to a place in which the fabric of daily life was woven around care. According to Milligan (2000a), domestic space can be seen to have merged with a space for carrying out caring duties to become a 'site of caring'. In addition to this, many of the participants had to deal with various forms of care assistance inside the home, hence further facilitating the convergence of public and private within the home. Milligan argues that the restructuring of caring has resulted in an institutionalisation of the carer's private space (2000a: 55). Evidence of this was identified by some of the participants, who argued that they had to shape their daily lives by strict routine. This appeared to have been learned over time, and seemed to arise from the earlier years of rearing their child:

> He was hard to rear now I can assure you. We had to keep the doors locked. He used to walk around with nothing on, and he had no road sense. All he did all day was scream. I don't even know how I reared him. To be honest with you now. Only I had the patience, I said I suppose like with everything else, I had good patience with him. But anyway, you used to be running around looking for him. I was like Ronnie Delayney. (C22)

Coping with outside ableist assumptions can have severe implications on the carer *inside* the home. It can effect who comes and goes from the household. Furthermore, as carers argued, the rhythms and routines of the home are often re-organised to comfort the care recipient, including social activities, recreation, and administration. The homespace had changed from being relatively carefree to a careful monitoring of movement and traffic and noise. Some carers felt uncomfortable inviting neighbours, friends or other visitors inside the house because of the behaviour of their disabled adult. One of the most significant changes, according to Wiles (2003) was that the homespace is no longer a place for social entertaining. Carers may not have the energy to organise and entertain, or it is too difficult for the recipient, or the guests. This is more common with the presence of an adult with a profound level of autism in the home for example:

> Even visitors to the house is a big no no. Because he just goes crazy with new people. He gets very excitable. Not even new people. Even the grandparents. He doesn't like people invading his territory. I suppose he kinda wants us for himself. But he's kinda hyper. (C3)

Even when the care recipient had reached a large degree of independence, they often had few genuine friends. For the carer, this can be difficult to cope with, and highlights the significant transition from adolescence to adulthood for someone with an intellectual disability. This rite of passage which is marked by the leaving of school, and the beginning of a new period of independence, self-determination and autonomy, is made even starker when there is no network of friends to rely on:

> She's very independent. She has gone out in Dublin, out in Eddie Rockets [burger restaurant]. I suppose the one draw back is she doesn't have her own pals. She's very independent though. If she's here by herself, she would be perfectly happy to sit and watch tv, playstation…she's ok. I suppose the one draw back is she doesn't have her own pals. She doesn't really have her own friends. People do ring her, for general chit-chat but I'd never hear her say, 'how about the cinema tonight?' I'd like to hear that. She had her brother and sister in school, so she had their friends. (C17)

Altogether then, the private space of the home can be a very different space, than that of an able-bodied family. It can be one characterised by isolation, loneliness and imbued with different social meanings. This offers a different perspective of the home as a therapeutic space for the family caregiver. While it can potentially contribute to the well-being of a young adult with an intellectual disability, for caregivers the home as a therapeutic landscape operates more as a goal (Williams, 2002), in which coping strategies, routines and restrictions have to be applied. From the perspective of the caregivers, the extent to which the home operates as a therapeutic landscape for them is questionable.

Developing Wider Hidden Geographies

As a result of the many challenges carers and their disabled adult children face in public life, and the interrelated dependence on their homespace, isolation was always a significant threat. Indeed, for some, the common bond of care-giving was the sense of isolation that comes from living outside the 'norm'. On a personal level, a carer may have little available time for social interaction with friends and with neighbours, or even with those members of the family outside the household or the immediate vicinity:

> You could live in inner city Dublin in a multi-storey block of flats and as a carer you are as isolated from the rest of the world as some people living on a mountainside with the nearest aid being 10 miles away. You are as hidden in the community as they are because you are left, and abandoned and on your own. (CO4)

For this reason, most families had invested much time on developing networks of 'safe havens' (Pinfold, 2000). These often took the form of natural (informal) supports within the family's personal network, such as supportive neighbours and friends, which the family had developed a relationship with:

> If we're going away anywhere, our next door neighbour here, she's brilliant. And [Orla] regards her as a second mother. Anytime we go away on holidays all she has to do is go in there. And she sleeps and all. Which is great. It eases your mind. (C20)

Often support like this can be much more flexible, inexpensive and can sometimes offer more assurance for carers than 'formal' services from the state. Consequently, key sites like other families' homes who had a child with a disability, or a close connection with other families were agreed upon and etched out in their maps of use where both felt comfortable in terms of attitudinal repose. In the words of one carer:

> In reality what you need to do is develop extended families as such. For example, if you had a friendship, or relationship with [James] or a person with a disability and you found it comfortable for [James] to come to you. And you also found it comfortable to go to them. So they're looked upon as a visitor or friend. And I think that's the model to develop (C3).

This example was quite common for carers, where they found that taking the care recipient to another family's homes, where both could feel comfortable, worked well for their own caring position. However, most contact between neighbours occurs informally and the extent of neighbourly aid can vary hugely from case to case. Variations in the social contact and aid-giving between neighbours is by and large due to a number of factors including: proximity of residence; duration of residence at a particular address and within a town; length of time of acquaintance; common workplace or work experience; common church membership; common life-cycle situation; and family ties or connections (Cecil et al., 1987).

In addition to these grass-roots safe havens, there are also opportunities to get support from the day activities organised by the local nonprofit service providers. Being associated with local disability service providers often meant that families were linked in with local activities such as 'special' drama groups, sport clubs, and social outings. Other examples of safe havens would be local parents' organisations which are grass-roots voluntary groups organised and ran by parents of people with intellectual disabilities, who share their own time and resources to create day support and indirectly respite for the parents:

> She loves going to the club, [Parents Together]. That's the reason we're involved in the club. Well [Joan] has been more involved on that particular one. But we're founding members of the club [Parents Together]. And that was through

> [Corporation Dublin], which would have been part of Bertie Ahern's [Irish PM] branch of that. He put money into that to set up groups to target people on the peripheries. Funding became available, and from that now [Joan] is the treasurer. It's going well financially, and it's going well in terms of the activities that they have for the kids, and the adults – we get them out to the beauticians, we get them out for meals, to get them bowling. And it's a matter of dropping [our daughter] down to the club, and she went off with her peers, so she wasn't with us.
>
> *And that gives respite to you?*
>
> Course it does. And it is independent living too. That branch of it comes into it too. (C7)

This description of a local parent's organisation by one of the carers shows the importance these groups can play in the local community. Moreover, the expression that it *is* independent living too, despite being exclusively with and *for* people with disabilities, demonstrates families' perceptions that activities do not need to be unequivocally 'mainstream' to be independent; rather, many carers felt the person can be independent *within* the safe spaces of collective communities. While these safe havens all represent an extension of the carer's narrow geographies beyond the homespace, at the same time, these spaces demonstrate a complex hidden geography, at the margins of mainstream public life. This could be perceived as leading to increased marginalisation into ever smaller spaces, on the 'outer fringes of the daily round' (Laws and Radford, 1998: 99). For this reason, many disability advocates argue that these are spaces of exclusion, given their sole disability focus. However, geographers such as Hall (2005) are calling for a re-appraisal of these spaces. He argues that the situations and experiences of exclusion/inclusion are complex and 'entangled'.

While it is important to identify and challenge the underlying reasons for and processes of the social exclusion of people with intellectual disabilities, at the same time, it would be a mistake to be unreservedly critical of familes acting collectively and providing opportunities for building a supportive, inclusive and empowering 'stretched community' (Valentine, 2001, cited in Hall, 2005) of people with intellectual disabilities and their supporters. Given the threat of isolation mentioned at the start of this section, it was clear that the parents were attempting to develop a wider 'caringspace' or therapeutic landscape, stretching the ethic of care across multiple sites in their local community. In these places, the person with intellectual disabilities could learn to assert their own needs and identities rather than cope with everyday exclusionary experiences in 'mainstream' public life. In this way, this local landscape of care is remapped to incorporate these secure spaces. Given that changing societal behaviour to be more 'accommodating' remains recalcitrant, these coping strategies remain an important part of the lives of carers and their adult children. Moreover, government and service providers still have an important role to continue to provide support and widen these caringscapes over the visible mainstream spaces that continue to exclude.

Conclusion

The impact of caring, reflected in the mobility and routine of carers' lives at the level of the body, the homespace, and the public and hidden community, all showed signs of inter-related physical, social, and emotional aspects. In caring for an adult with an intellectual disability in particular, these situations were driven by intense emotions. According to Wiles (2003), caregiving work is as much emotional and social as it is physical. These emotions, such as discomfort, guilt, fear and so on, had strong spatial effects, as seen in the restrictions on carers' daily geographies. A major cause of these emotions was having to care for a 'representative' body, which involved dealing with the representation of the disabled body in society and having to challenge the barriers caused by these social attitudes. This aspect of care work was just as important, if not more so, than the physical tasks.

Because many carers are restricted spatially, the focus of everyday life had largely become the homespace. As a result, the homespace had changed a great deal. The household had become firstly imbued with different meanings and secondly was characterised by different daily patterns and routines. One of their strategies for coping was in many cases the imposition of spatial constraints on themselves and the care recipient. The research on care highlights the fact that space and scale are therefore important issues in understanding the caring situation.

Carers' experiences of getting outside the household and using public spaces revealed how the caring experience is one that is embedded in relationships with social 'norms' of behaviour. Feeling 'out-of-place' was a common experience for the carer, especially in busy public places, where there was less patience on the part of the public. Again, many had developed coping strategies or had overcome feelings of discomfort. However, many also still talked about being very susceptible to becoming socially isolated as well as being physically isolated within the home.

Social and affective support outside the family tended to come from those in a similar situation to themselves. Many carers had developed networks through parents' groups and neighbours which reciprocally provided support for individuals with disabilities in their community. These networks of 'safe havens' offer families the potential to widen their circle of support, which often provides more sustainable and encouraging forms of care.

Chapter 9
Conclusion

The research which underpinned this book has come from a range of sources including archival and policy research, other academic texts, and interviews with service providers, carer associations and carers. The book is structured in three related parts, and the content makes a progression from the macro to micro scales. It firstly explores the key concepts around landscapes of care, specifically family care, welfare and citizenship as they apply to families of adults with intellectual disabilities, and offers broad critiques and theorisation around these. Next, it examines English, US and Irish approaches to the provision of welfare as they apply to carers and disabled adults. This shows how historical developments reflect changing perceptions of the role of the family and particularly women, and of individual rights over time. Alongside this, it examines the ways in which the structures and values of government itself can shape perceptions of carers and individuals with intellectual disabilities, and responses to the needs of each. The final section focuses specifically on the Irish example, by undertaking a closer inspection of contemporary provision of care and the experiences of carers in this system.

The book seeks to address the difficult tension between the needs and rights of adults with intellectual disabilities and the needs and rights of those who care for them often on an unpaid or 'lay' basis. This central issue, along with the illustration of the deeply contextual and historical nature of 'landscapes of care' serves to unpack the interconnections between broader discussions on care, and the local, 'household' level experiences of caregivers themselves. It thus provides a nuanced and powerful illustration of the inter-relationship between space, place and politics at these different scales.

This concluding chapter discusses the contributions of this book as a whole, to our understandings of caregiving and the landscapes of support which underpins it. It outlines in more detail these contributions under three main headings: the discursive role of welfare regimes, Ireland's welfare approach in comparison with England and the US, and carers' lives and identities. Drawing from the theoretical framework of the book, under each of these headings, it assesses what can be drawn from the interpretation of the principal findings. In the final section, the main limitations of the book and suggestions for further research are discussed.

The Discursive Role in Welfare Regimes

This book was primarily concerned with understanding different family carer policies and services in an international context. From a disciplinary perspective, despite the emergence of a large number of studies examining home care, this study makes a broader cross-national comparison of carer support services, and the ideologies underlying them. The case studies of care support for people with intellectual disabilities in England and the US, in comparison to Ireland, have shown how the social, economic, and political histories have had different geographical consequences on family carers. At the root of this was how citizenship rights and the welfare state targeted carers. The initial phase of the research looked at these concepts of citizenship and rights. It was argued that unlike civil and political rights, the notion of social rights has given rise to much contestation within the interactions of governance, as this is the field where collective-bargaining, clientalism, and constructions of what is 'in the national interest' are played out. In other words, this is the specific site where the participation of different actors intersect to enable the discourses surrounding carers to feed into policy.

While budgetary constraints have and continue to be a cause of concern for governments, the construction of social discourse is still key in determining how the resources should be redistributed in society. While it is clear that each country constructs different institutional barriers and processes of redistribution, it is also clear that rights and responsibilities are more fundamental concerns in the public's consciousness, and feed directly into how the government should divide their resources. More specifically, the notion of the rights and responsibilities of carers and how well they were identified in each state fundamentally shaped the responsiveness of community care policy. Underpinning many of the differences in welfare states, there is a dominant welfare discourse which continues to construct disabled people as dependent and therefore in need of care, despite the fact that bodies like the UN insist that disability is a matter of human rights (Arnadottir and Quinn, 2009).

This book has offered an exploration into how nations construct the identity of the carer, and the spatial implications of such a construction. A general difference in social attitudes and welfare ideologies clearly had implications on the way carers are supported by the State. Throughout the case study chapters, the analysis pinpointed acts of legislation, as it was through these that the changes in social discourses were most visible. In order to understand the conditions under which our present way of thinking and acting upon carers has taken shape and to make intelligible the naturalisation and normalisation of their socially fashioned identities, it was important to understand the diversity and complexity of the processes of self-formation, and 'the interconnection between self-formation and political and governmental processes and practices' (Dean 1994: 145). The post-structuralist theoretical framework allowed for the analysis of the social construction of disability and care which triggered this policy, and shaped how policies changed over time. This builds on academic literature in disability and care by looking critically at how the discourses around these issues have led to these distinct material effects. At the same time as analysing the political-economy in each country, the research examined the ideological environment that developed over time – characterised by disability lobby groups, carer groups, the Church, wider civil society and so on – all of which helped shape notions of rights, needs, and entitlement in each country. Moreover, their perspectives also shaped the identity of carers and disabled citizens in the mainstream. In each case, the discourses fed into different material effects, as seen in the different welfare states and community care policy.

In terms of looking abroad, it has been clear that the construction of social 'norms' within the different jurisdictions regarding the role of family and disability has led to quite distinct local practices. Although there was a common objective in all countries to maintain the dignity and independence of the adult with the intellectual disability in their own homes, the assumptions regarding the responsibility of family differed greatly in each country. As a result carers were directly and indirectly affected by a huge range of different acts of legislation and restructuring policy in such areas as family policy, disability legislation, health care restructuring, community care policy as well as budgetary targets. Each of these have material and institutional effects and are premised on the discourses, ideologies, and interactions in the state at a particular time.

In the US, in the early 1800s, caregivers of disabled siblings were depicted as dedicated, loving, and spiritually improved by their labours. Being intellectually disabled did not disqualify people from work, education, social invitations, or travel. However, with the rise of social Darwinism as a powerful scientific discourse from the mid-19th century onwards came the elaborate process of establishing disability as 'the Other'. The learned reasoning changed to believe that parents of 'idiots' were diseased and sinful, and they began to experience increasing shame and despair as the century passed (Richards, 2004). The dilemma of rearing a dependent sibling in a society grounded in values of independence and competition has haunted US family caregivers over the course of two centuries (Brockley, 2004). However, with the rise of civil rights and the disability movement after World War Two, disability became a category under which the State had to afford rights. Indirectly family caregivers were given support under the *Americans with Disabilities Act* (ADA) in 1990, which marked a milestone in the struggle for the basic civil rights of people with disabilities.

While the discourses and policy at Federal level maintain the ideals of capitalism and independence, at the State level much of the policies are interconnected with local notions of need. The changing context of US history has clearly shaped how best each State has dealt with family caregivers. Although there has been the recent establishment of the National Family Caregiver Support Program at the federal level, progress in caregiver policy is clearly a contested terrain at the state level, as some states feel the family caregiver should be supported more directly than others. More generally, the landscape of care in the US has typically constructed the care recipient as the target of social support.

In England, the recognition of the family carer and their needs in mainstream society has led to an altogether different material support system. While their policies have altered with the changing economic, social, and political context of England, the spotlight on rights and independence of the care recipient has not been as dominant as in the US. The belief in the ability of the welfare state to ameliorate the problems for intellectually disabled people constructed a landscape of care which naturalised the role of the family in sustaining their independence much more clearly. With this came an equally elaborate community support system to the US, however, and one which has more noticeably targeted the carer. While carers in England get more recognition in political discourse, it is more difficult to qualitatively judge across England and the US which is the better system for carers. The US rights movement has arguably focused on the more vociferous, young physically disabled population, while those with intellectual disabilities have been hampered from the US values of independence and competition. For this reason, parents of adult children with intellectual disabilities have arguably found it harder under this model. In England, while the extension of rights towards disabled people has not stretched as far, the reliance on the welfare state and community support for intellectually disabled adults has arguably better served carers. However, while the English welfare state has produced both benefits and problems, and such policies are only beginning to empower carers, for the most part, the English landscape of care does offer a more comprehensive support network unlike the US or Ireland.

Ireland's Welfare Approach

The book has offered a fundamental examination of the spatial structures of caring in Irish society. This has incorporated looking at the wider caring community and examined access to caring sites outside the home. In contrast to England and the US, Ireland developed an ad hoc approach to supporting and empowering carers. In general, having someone with a disability in the family still remains a 'personal tragedy', as a result of the long-standing charity based model which emerged from the limited involvement of the State. An extensive voluntary sector is now funded and loosely managed by the State and has been complimented by some statutory payments and a largely voluntary community care workforce. Welfare in Ireland, far from promoting social integration, has retained a large category of unassisted carers, generally isolated and excluded.

The discourses from the Church and the early free State constructed a very firm notion of the family being the cornerstone of society. Over the course of the last century, family carers have been left with little or no support as a result of the State's reluctance to 'interfere' with the family. While Eugenics and social Darwinism never became dominant in Ireland, there were nevertheless huge rates of institutionalisation for both 'idiots' and the 'insane'. With a lack of rights or regulatory supports, care outside of the institution was largely neglected and isolating. Historically, having such a child in the family was automatic grounds for exclusion. For the most part, this situation did not improve until the 1960s. This change came from social pressure to de-institutionalise and move to community care. The State started to fund some charity and voluntary agencies. However, progress in community care only gathered pace in the late 1990s with the economic boom, the weakening of the Church's position in society, and the increasing influence of the EU. This led to increased funding of the sector and the introduction of some means-tested benefits. Despite these provisions the landscape of care in Ireland is still in its infancy. Investment in welfare and health care has largely been catch-up funding in infrastructure and services.

As a result, many families find themselves in positions of powerless dependency. Because home help and carer support is poorly managed and subject to fluctuating budgetary levels, many families often consider themselves lucky if they receive a wraparound 'cradle to grave' adult service. While these may represent a secure option for families and their child, in reality, they have the potential to further disconnect young adults with intellectual disabilities from their communities and break down the natural supports which neighbours and friends can offer within a circle of support. While the situation is improving, there is a general lack of shared knowledge between service providers, and support can be largely ad hoc and under-funded.

While there have been some recent improvements, such as increases in the Carer's Allowance, discursively, carers are still framed in Catholic-conservative notions of child-rearing with limited social support, despite having an intellectually disabled child. Social Work in general does not have family carers in its remit, tending to focus on issues with 'problem families' such as drug use and delinquency. Ireland has therefore failed to provide the strength of civil and social rights, accorded to US citizens, or the range of community support and civil protections offered to English citizens. Instead, Ireland offers a limited unsystematic blend of tightly-regulated State supports and weak social rights. Moreover, these are fragmented across scale, and reliant on local political guarantees. By international standards, the landscape of care for carers of intellectually disabled adults in Ireland serve as a unique case-study of how different ideologies can limit and hamper support systems for different groups.

Carer's Lives and Identities

Another strong contribution of the research concerns the development of the geographical 'lifeworld' of carers of young adults with intellectual disabilities. Given the earlier section's focus on international comparative carer support models, the latter focus on the local lives of carers provides a glimpse at the inter-relationship between national level state policies and attitudes towards the role of carers of adult children with intellectual disabilities and the experiences of carers themselves.

It was clear when looking at carer's lives, that the service system beyond the household shapes both the daily practices within the home, but also the way in which parents embody the role of carer. In Foucault's analysis, people's actions and meanings are shaped by discursive and non-discursive forces that flow through the positions they inhabit (Danaher et al., 2000: 103). Importantly carer solidarity is discursively as well as materially constructed and a carer 'identity' is shaped by many other discourses of identity and social differentiation. The carers' narratives revealed how the impacts of the state are significant in every possible dimension of their lives, to the extent that caregiving comes to dominate every experience; emotional, physical and spatial. For carers, the home is the major site of exploitation; the locus where class and gender and other ideologies intersect. Public economic discourse increasingly invades this personal and private space, hailing carers as either causes or co-victims of economic stagnation and instability.

Further, the inter-connections between broader discussions on care at the comparative scale and family lives at the local, offers a nuanced and powerful illustration of the general argument that space, place and politics are inter-related. It demonstrates the connection between different scales (household, national, international) and situated historical context. This multi-scalar analysis also allows for an examination of the possible ways in which the idea of therapeutic landscapes can inform the debates in caregiving by relocating some of that discussion into the everyday worlds of both paid and unpaid carers of adults with intellectual disabilities and those adults themselves along with the political-institutional arrangements to support them.

As evidenced in recent critiques of therapeutic landscapes (see Gastaldo et al. 2004), traditional ways in which the concept has been used often failed to adequately inform or explain the ways in which individuals construct and use these landscapes. Moreover, Wilson (2003) criticises the failure to acknowledge that therapeutic landscapes may be individualised, everyday, dispersed, unbounded and intricately constructed. Clearly, the 'caring spaces' illustrated through the family narratives offers a more nuanced elucidation of the multiple and complex ways in which individuals must construct 'safe havens' for their sons or daughters with disabilities. The latter chapters thus build on a small body of research that has been focused on the ways in which therapeutic landscapes are created, reproduced and negotiated by marginalised groups, for example, people with mental health problems (Geores and Gesler, 1999; Parr, 1999). In the same way, carers of young adults with disabilities must employ routines and coping strategies to create, reproduce and negotiate therapeutic spaces of well-being.

Ultimately, living *within* a landscape of care is characterised by the proximity of the carer to the outside environment, made up of agents, policies, and services that seek to shape it. As identified in the last chapter, proximity affects the likelihood, nature and intensity of providing care (Wiles, 2003). Despite the unique nature of individual caregiving experiences, each carer has to grapple with a shared mainstream discursive and ideological construction of their identity as well as the material consequences of these discourses in the everyday care services (characterised by different benefits, entitlement rules, service philosophies and so on). Lash and Urry's (1987) work on the significance of 'moorings', as sites and objects in which the irregularities of life latch on to, in order to provide a less-fluid process is helpful here. In other words, the hybridity of carers' lives are in a way 'latched on' to the service system. Being within a community care system with rules and regulations which tied carers into various positions often undermined the hybridity of everyday life. It was also evident from carers' experiences, that there is still a strong notion of the 'social contract', in that not caring properly breaches the social contract and society as a whole is the victim. In this way, it operates as a 'self-steering mechanism' (Foucault, 1986). As a result, often carers are reluctant to ask for help, and social services tend to assume carers are coping fine until they tell them otherwise. Carers are often the last people to voice their concerns, despite often suffering from above-average levels of loneliness, depression and loss of income (Douglas and Philpot, 1998).

At the same time however, this 'social contract' is not a hegemonic imposing form of power. Different coping strategies by carers highlight the fact that rule following is always to some degree discretionary, elaborative, ad hoc. Foucault (1979: 95–6) himself argued that:

> Resistance is integral to power. The existence of power relationships depends on a multiplicity of points of resistance which are the odd terms in relations of power; they are inscribed in the latter as irreducible opposite.

In Gibson-Graham's (1996) terms, despite being homogeneously theorised by structural or hegemonic conceptions, the forms of resistance taken by carers take multiple and diverse forms in everyday local contexts as well as at the national 'carer representative' level. Their individual struggles with exploitation are an ever-present experience with significant (though not unidirectional) transformative effects. These take the form of confronting health and social services, by-passing bureaucratic barriers by contacting local political representatives, lobbying government for change, and confronting public reactions. These practices serve to highlight the fluid and dynamic nature of caregiving, and the intertwining of the political, social and economic discourses and material practices and the individual carer's daily lives.

A post-structural approach, consequently, provides an effective tool through which to examine how carers and care recipients are socially constructed across space and place, and how the discourses have manifested themselves in the landscape of care support. It also shows that despite the presence of formal legislation, often social perceptions and personal attitudes at the local scale remain significantly relevant in how carers access everyday services. By analysing both the historical development of welfare in Ireland and how carers were perceived, and the current experiences of carers within this system, the approach was able to highlight how the traditional portrayal of carers as 'women in their place' has led to a deeply contextual landscape of care in which national, local and embodied scales are closely inter-connected.

Limitations and Suggestions for Further Research

The conclusions which can be drawn from this book provide several leads for further research. In this section, any shortcomings of the research are acknowledged, and an agenda for future research identified.

The methodology chosen for the book was dependent on the two central research questions, firstly, how does Ireland's model of care compare with that of England and the US, and secondly how care within this model is experienced on the ground. Methodologically, the tension between the scale of a cross-country analysis and a local analysis in Ireland proved a challenge. By developing a research design that incorporated an extensive literature review of primary and secondary data, complemented by interviews with key actors, the book was able to develop a cohesive collection of contextual data at the national level. However, it was not possible within the confines of this book, due to methodological issues of time and resource constraints, to examine, in depth, the local experiences of care in England and the US. Thus the comparative chapters failed to illustrate in any great depth, the experience of the lifeworld of carers and of the actors within community care in these countries. To complement the present research, future studies might focus more on linking the histories of care support to more in-depth qualitative analysis in each country to provide more specific comparisons between 'the experiences of care' in different countries.

Secondly, in the search for an explanation of the geography of community care in Ireland, the research investigated the experiences of voluntary groups, health services and carers. This data uncovered general supply and access issues of health and community care services, as well as how services are configured; in short, how they are provided. However, the methodology failed to show a national surface identification of patterns of geographical inequality in the provision and utilisation of community care services. Thus, while the interview data did provide a detailed description of the landscape of care, a more systematic and extensive quantitative inventory and visualisation, including GIS mapping of carers and services, would complement the views and experiences of family carers in each area. A mapping of services would clearly have beneficial planning applications and provide more immediate geographical comparisons between administrative regions.

Finally, while broader disability policy has an impact on adults with intellectual disabilities, it is harder to make generalisations from this one category of disability to the wider disability population. Furthermore, while carers of the elderly and physically disabled use much of the same service structure, the findings of the study do not directly relate to, or are easily generalised to, the wider population. Further research is required in order to replicate this approach for these other carers. Thus, the present case study serves as one element in a broader academic process of care research. A linking of the kind of care experiences by other carers, and from other regions, with a spatial depiction of services, would make an important contribution to the academic and policy debate on caring for carers.

Bibliography

Abberley, P. 1987 The concept of oppression and the development of a social theory of disability. *Disability, Handicap and Society*. 2(1), 5–19.

Abrams, P. 1978. *Neighbourhood Care and Social Policy*. Berkhamsted: Volunteer Centre.

Acton, G. 2002. Health-Promoting Self-Care in Family Caregivers. *Western Journal of Nursing Research*, 24(1), 73–86.

Amnesty International. 2003. *Mental Illness: The Neglected Quarter: A report by Amnesty International. Irish Section. Promoting the rights of the one in four people affected by mental illness in Ireland*, http://www.amnesty.ie/netw/mentalhealth/3%20Community%20care.pdf. February [accessed 29 September 2006].

Anderson, J.M. 1990. Home care management in chronic illness and the self-care movement: An analysis of ideologies and economic processes influencing policy decisions. *Advances in Nursing Science* 12(2), 71–83.

Anderson, M. and Rosenberg, M.W. 1990. Ontario's Underserviced Area Program revisited: An indirect analysis, *Social Science and Medicine*, 30(1), 35–44.

Arber, S. and Gilbert, N. 1989. Transitions in caring: gender, life course and care of the elderly. In *Becoming and Being Old: Sociological Approaches to Later Life*, edited by B. Bytheway, T. Keil, P. Allatt and A. Bryman. London: Sage.

Arber, S. and Ginn, J. 1999. Gender Differences in Informal Caring. In *The Sociology of the Family: A Reader* edited by G. Allan. Oxford: Blackwell.

Arnadottir, O. and Quinn, G. 2009. *The UN Convention on the Rights of Persons With Disabilities: European and Scandinavian Perspectives*. New York: Brill Publishers.

Arno, P.S., Levine, C. and Memmott, M.M. 1999. The Economic Value of Informal Caregiving: President Clinton's proposal to provide relief to family caregivers opens a long-overdue discussion of this 'invisible' health care sector. *Health Affairs* 18(2), 182–8.

Arskey, H. 2002. Rationed Care: Assessing the Support Needs of Informal Carers in English Social Services Authorities. *Journal of Social Policy* 31(1), 81–101.

Atkin, K. 1992. Similarities and differences between informal carers. In *Carers: Research and practice*, edited by J. Twigg. London: HMSO, 30–58.

Atkinson, D. 1997. *An Auto/biographical Approach to Learning Disability Research*. Aldershot: Ashgate.

Ayer, S. and Alaszewski, A. 1984. *Community Care and the Mentally Handicapped: Services for Mothers and Their Mentally Handicapped Children*. London: Croom Helm.

Balibar, E. 1995. 'Culture and Identity'. In *The Identity in Question*, edited by J. Rajchman. New York: Routledge.

Bandman, B. 1973. *Do Children Have Any Natural Rights?* Proceedings of the 29th Annual General Meeting of the Philosophy of Education Society, 234–42.

Barclay Report. 1982. *Social Workers: Their Role and Tasks*. London: Bedford Square Press.

Barnes, M. 1997. *Care, Communities and Citizens*. New York: Longman.

Baron, S., Riddell, S., and Wilkinson, H. 1998. The best burgers? The person with learning difficulties as worker, in *The Disability Reader: Social Science Perspectives*, edited by T. Shakespeare. London: Cassell.

Barrington, R. 1987. *Health, Medicine and Politics in Ireland, 1900–1970*. Dublin: Institute of Public Administration.

Bartlett, P. and Wright, D. 1999. *Outside the Walls of the Asylum: The History of Care in the Community 1750–2000*. London: Athlone Press.

Batavia, A. 2003. *Independent Living: A Viable Option for Long-term Care*. Clearwater, Florida: ABI Professional Publications.

Baxter, C., Poonia, K., Ward, L., et al. 1990. *Double Discrimination: Issues and Services for People with Learning Difficulties from Black and Ethnic Minority Communities*. London: King's Fund Centre/Commission for Racial Equality.

BBC News. 1999. *The origins of community care*, 13 October, http://news.bbc.co.uk/1/hi/health/229517.stm [accessed 12 August, 2003].

Berven H.M. and Blanck, P.D. 1998. The Economics of the Americans With Disabilities Act Part II – Patents and Innovations in Assistive Technology, *Journal of Law, Ethics and Public Policy*, 12(9), 9–120.

Beveridge, W. 1942. *Social Insurance and Allied Services*. Beveridge Report, Cmd 6404. London: HMSO.

Bhabba, H.K. 1994. *The Location of Culture*. London: Routledge.

Biscay, M. 1999. *The Glorious Revolution of 1688*, http://www.skyminds.net/civilization/03_glorious_revolution_of_1688.php. [accessed 24 August, 2004].

Blakemore, K. and Drake, R.F. 1996. *Understanding Equal Opportunity Policies*. London: Prentice Hall.

Bloy, M. 2002. *The 1601 Elizabethan Poor Law*, http://www.victorianweb.org/history/poorlaw/elizpl.html [accessed 30 July 2004].

Bond, D. and Conniffe, D. 2002. *Cross-Regional Equity in Health Care Funding*, Working Paper Series, National Institute for Regional and Spatial Analysis, 3 January 2002.

Bourdieu, P. 1991. *Language and Symbolic Power*. Cambridge, MA: Harvard University Press.

Bowers, F. 2005. *Health Board overhaul – or just smoke and mirrors?* http://www.irishhealth.com/?level=4&id=4555 [accessed 24 April 2005].

Boyd, D. and Nathan, R.P. 2003. The Current State Fiscal Crisis and its Aftermath. September, Washington, D.C.: The Henry J. Kaiser Family Foundation.

Brain Injury Resource Foundation. 2003. *Lifespan Respite Care Act of 2003*, http://www.birf.info/artman/publish/article_308.shtml [accessed 10 March 2005].

Brennan, D. 2004. Commentary: A consideration of the social trajectory of psychiatric nursing in Ireland. *Journal of Psychiatric and Mental Health Nursing* 11, 494–501.

Brennan, P. 1979. Women in revolt, *Magill*, 2. 7 April, pp. 34–6.

Brockley, J. 2004. Martyred Mothers and Merciful Fathers: Exploring Disability and Motherhood in the Lives of Jerome Greenfield and Raymond Repouille, in *Mental Retardation in America*, edited by S. Noll, and J. Trent Jr. New York: New York University Press, 293–312.

Brody, E. 1981. 'Women in the Middle' and family help to older people. *The Gerontologist* 21: 471–9.

Bulmer, M. 1987. *The Social Basis of Community Care*. London: Allen and Unwin.

Burns, M.E. 2009 Medicaid Managed Care and Health Care Access for Adult Beneficiaries with Disabilities, *Health Services Research.* 44(5), 1521–41.

Busfield, J. 1986. *Managing Madness: Changing Ideas and Practice*. London: Unwin Hyman Ltd.

Butler, R. and Bowley, S. 1997. Bodies in Space: an exploration of disabled people's experience of public space. *Environment and Planning D: Society and Space*. 14, 414–31.

Byrkjeflot, H. and Neby, S. 2008. The end of the decentralised model of healthcare governance? Comparing developments in the Scandinavian hospital sectors. *Journal of Health Organisation and Management*, 22(4), 331–49.

Bytheway, B. and Johnson, J. 2008. The Social Construction of Carers, in *Understanding Health and Social Care: An Introductory Reader,* edited by J. Johnson and C. De Souza. London: Polity Press.

Cantwell, J. 2001. Long Term Care Insurance: Sooner Rather than Later, in *Who Will Pay for Long Term Care?: Insights from the Partnership Programs,* edited by N. McCall. Chicago: Health Administration Press, 263–71.

Carewatch. 2004. *Carewatch Care Services UK Franchise*, http://www.whichfranchise.com/franchisorPage.cfm?companyID=2138 [accessed 20 June 2004].

Carter, R. 1995. *Helping Yourself Help Others: A Book for Caregivers*. New York: Three Rivers Press.

Case, G.S.B., Himmelstein, D.U. and Woolhandler, S. 2002. No Care for the Caregivers: Declining Health Insurance Coverage for Health Care Personnel and their Children, 1988–1998. *American Journal of Public Health* 92(3), 404–9.

Castles, F.G. 2004. *The Future of the Welfare State: Crisis Myths and Crisis Realities*. Oxford: Oxford University Press.

Cecil, R., Offer, J. and Leger, F.S. 1987. *Informal Welfare: A Sociological Study of Care in Northern Ireland.* Suffolk: Paradigm Print.

Census Bureau. 1996. *Survey of Income and Program Participation*. Washington, D.C.

Central Statistics Office. 2004. Disability and Carers. Dublin: Government of Ireland.

Chappell, N.L. Reid, R.C. and Dow, E. 2001. Respite reconsidered: A typology of meanings based on the caregiver's point of view, *Journal of Aging Studies*. 15(2), 201–16.

Charlton, J. 1998. *Nothing About Us Without Us: Disability Oppression and Empowerment*. Berkeley, CA: University of California Press.

Chartier, D.R. 1999. *Roosevelt's 'New Deal'*, http://www.newdeallegacy.org/history_newdeal.html [accessed 24 July 2008].

Chatterjee, L. and Mitra, M. 1998. Evolution of federal and state policies for persons with disability in the United States: Efficiency and welfare impacts. *The Annals of Regional Science* 32, 347–65.

Christie, N. 1989. *Beyond Loneliness and Institutions: Communes for Extraordinary People*. Oslo: Norwegian University Press.

Clarke, J., Cochrane, A. and Smart, C. 1987. *Ideologies of Welfare: From Dreams to Disillusionment*. London: Hutchinson.

Clarke, J. and Langan, M. 2001a. The British Welfare State: Foundation and Modernization. In *Comparing Welfare States: Britain in International Context*, edited by A. Cochrane, and J. Clarke. London: Sage, in association with the Open University.

Clarke, J. and Langan, M. 2001b. Restructuring Welfare: The British Welfare Regime in the 1980s. In *Comparing Welfare States: Britain in International Context*, edited by A. Cochrane, and J. Clarke. London: Sage, in association with the Open University.

Clarke, J., Cochrane, A. and Gewirtz, S. (eds). 2001. *Comparing Welfare States*. 2nd edition. London: Sage.

Close, P. 1995. State Care, Control and Contradictions. In *The State and Caring*, edited by P. Close. London: Macmillan.

Cochrane, A. and Clarke, J. (eds). 2001. *Comparing Welfare States: Britain in International Context*. London: Sage, in association with the Open University.

Comhairle. 2001. The Community and Voluntary Sector. *Relate* August 28(11), 1–9.

Comhairle. 2002. Supporting Carers: A Social Policy Report. July, Dublin: Comhairle.

Commission on the Family. 1998. *Strengthening Families For Life*. Final Report to the Minister for Social, Community and Family Affairs. July 1998, Dublin.

Commission on the Status of People with Disabilities. 1996. A Strategy for Equality, Dublin.

Commission for Social Care Inspection, 2004. Performance Rating For Social Services in England. November. Department for Health. UK Government.

Comptroller and Auditor General (C&AG). 2005. Value for Money Review: Provision of Disability Services by Nonprofit Organisations. Report No. 52. December 2005. Dublin: Stationery Office.

Comptroller and Auditor General (C&AG). 2008. *Annual Report on the Accounts of the Public Services – 2007*. September. Dublin: Stationery Office.

Condorcet, M. 1795. *Sketch for a Historical Picture of the Progress of the Human Mind.*

Conroy, J. 1996. *Outcomes of Robert Wood Johnston Foundation's National Initiative on Self-Determination for Persons with Developmental Disabilities Final Report on 3 Years of Research and Analysis*. Narberth, PA: Center for Outcome Analysis.

Conroy, J., Fullerton, A., Brown, M., and Garrow, J. 2002. *Outcomes of the Robert Wood Johnson Foundation's National Initiative on Self-Determination for Persons with Developmental Disabilities: Final Report on 3 Years of Research and Analysis*. December. Narberth, PA: Center for Outcome Analysis.

Coppock, V. and Hopton, J. 2000. From care in the community to care by the community, *Critical Perspectives on Mental Health*, 1(3), 40–44.

Cousins, M. 1995. *The Irish Social Welfare System in Ireland.* Dublin: The Round Hall Press Ltd.

Cranford, C., Fudge, J., Tucker, E. and Vosko, L.F. 2005. *Self Employed Workers Organize: Law, Policy and Unions*. Ontario: McGill-Queens University Press.

Creese, G. 2006. Government Restructuring and Non-Profit Settlement Agencies in Vancouver: Bringing Advocacy Back In. In *Landscapes of Voluntarism: New Spaces of Health, Welfare and Governance*, edited by D. Conradson and C. Milligan. London: The Policy Press, 191–209.

Crookshank, F.G. 1924. *The Mongol in Our Midst: A Study of Man and His Three Faces.* London: Kegan Paul.

Cuellar, N. and Butts, J.B. 1999. Caregiver Distress: What Nurses in Rural Settings Can Do to Help. *Nursing Forum* 34(3), 24–30.

Cummins, S., Curtis, S., Diez-Roux, A.V. and Macintyre, S. 2007. Understanding and representing 'place' in health research: a relational approach. *Social Science and Medicine*, 65(9), 1825–38.

Curry, J. 1990. *Irish Social Services*. Institute of Public Administration, Dublin.

Dáil Éireann. 1997. Parliamentary Debates, Volume 481 – 9 October 1997, Written Answers – Residential Care. http://historical-debates.oireachtas.ie/D/0481/D.0481.199710090029.html. [accessed 7 October, 2004].

Dáil Éireann. 1989. Parliamentary Debates. Volume 387 – 1 March 1989. Ceisteanna – Questions. Oral Answers – National Council for the Aged Report, http://historical-debates.oireachtas.ie/D/0387/D.0387.198903010016.html [accessed 5 October, 2008].

Dale, P. 2003. Implementing the 1913 Mental Deficiency Act. *Social History of Medicine*, 16(3), 403–18.

Daly, A. and Walsh, D. 2002. Irish Psychiatric Hospitals and Units Census 2001. May. Dublin: Health Research Board.

Daly, M. 1989. *Women and Poverty*. Dublin: Attic Press/Combat Poverty Agency.

Daly, M. and Clavero, S. 2003. 'Contemporary Family Policy in Ireland and Europe'. School of Sociology and Social Policy. Belfast: Queen's University Press.

Daly, M. and Lewis, J. 2000. The concept of social care and the analysis of contemporary welfare, *British Journal of Sociology*. 51(2), 281–98.

Danaher, G., Schirato, T., and Webb, J. 2000. *Understanding Foucault*. London: Allen and Unwin.

Darwin, C. 1859. *The Origin of Species*, Available at: http://www.talkorigins.org/faqs/origin/introduction.html [accessed 15 February, 2010].

Deakin, N., Finer, C.J. and Matthews, B. 2004. *Welfare and the State: Critical Concepts in Political Science*. London: Routledge.

Dean, M. 1994. *Critical and Effective Histories: Foucault's Methods and Historical Sociology*. London: Routledge.

Dear, M., Wilton, R., Gaber, S L., Takahashi, L. 1997. Seeing people differently: the sociospatial construction of disability *Environment and Planning D: Society and Space* 15(4), 455–80.

Dear, M.J. and Wolch, J.R. 1987. *Landscapes of Despair: From Deinstitutionalisation to Homelessness*. Oxford: Polity Press.

Delanty, G. 2000. *Modernity and Postmodernity: Knowledge, Power and Self.* London: Sage.

Department of Health 1990. *Needs and Abilities: Report of the Review Group on Mental Handicap Services*, Dublin: Stationery Office.

Department of Health. 1980. *Report of the Working Party on Services for the Mentally Handicapped*. Dublin: Stationery Office.

Department of Health. 2000. The NHS Plan: A Plan for investment, a plan for reform. London: HMSO.

Department of Health. 2001. *Valuing People: A New Strategy for Learning Disability for the 21st Century*. London: HMSO.

Department of Health. 2005a. *National Service Frameworks*, http://www.dh.gov.uk/PolicyAndGuidance/HealthAndSocialCareTopics/HealthAndSocialCareArticle/fs/en?CONTENT_ID=4070951&chk=W3ar/W [accessed 21 February 2005].

Department of Health. 2005b. *Primary Care*, http://www.dh.gov.uk/PolicyAndGuidance/OrganisationPolicy/PrimaryCare/fs/en [accessed 22 February 2005].

Department of Health. 2009. *Valuing People Now: A New Three-Year Strategy for People with Learning Disabilities*. London: HMSO.

Department of Health and Children. DoHC. 1997. *Services to Persons with a Mental Handicap/Intellectual Disability: An Assessment of Need 1997–2001*. Dublin: Stationery Office.

Department of Health and Children. 2000. *Year 2000 Health Estimate: allocation to health breaks £4 billion barrier*, http://www.doh.ie/pressroom/pr19991111.html [accessed 24 May 2004].

Department of Health and Children. 2000. *A Framework for Supporting Voluntary Activity.* Dublin: Stationery Office.

Department of Health and Children. 2001. *Quality and Fairness – A Health System for You*. Dublin: Stationery Office.

Department of Health and Social Security. 1988. *The Griffiths Report: Community Care: Agenda for Action*. London: HMSO.

Department of Social Community and Family Affairs. 2001. *Changing for a Changing Ireland.* June 2001. Dublin: Stationery Office.

Department of Social Protection (formerly the Department of Social Community and Family Affairs). 2009. *Press Release: Government not proceeding with publication of a National Carer's Strategy*, 3 March 2009.

Department of Social Services. 1998. *Modernising Social Services*. London: HMSO.

Department of Social Services. 1998. *A New Contract for Welfare: New Ambitions for Our Country*. London: HMSO.

Derrida, J. 1991. *A Derrida Reader: Between the Blinds*. Brighton: Harvester Wheatsheaf.

Diamond, L., Blackfan, K.D., Baty, J.M. 1932. Erythroblastosis fetalis and its association with universal edema of the fetus, icterus gravis, neonatorum and anemia of the newborn. *J Pediatr*. 30, 269–309.

Diez-Roux, A.V. 2001. Investigating neighborhood and area effects on health, *American Journal Public Health*, 91(11), 1783–89.

Dinsmore, P. 2000. *The Origin of United States Welfare Model: A Comparison*, http://www.pitt.edu/~heinisch/ca_us.html. [accessed 1 June, 2007].

Disability Federation of Ireland. 2002. *An Overview of Irish Health Legislation*, www.wheel.ie/user/content/download/ 168/730/file/flac.pdf [accessed 16 September 2003].

Disability Federation of Ireland. 2009. *HSE Policy and Procedures for Funding Non-Statutory Organisations*, http://www.disability-federation.ie/index.php?uniqueID=175 [accessed 22 March 2010].

Disability Federation of Ireland. 2008. *Paper Submitted to the Joint Oireachtas Committee on Health and Children*, 1 July, 2008.

Disability Social History Project. 2003. *Disability History Timeline*, http://www.disabilityhistory.org/timeline_new.html [accessed 27 January 2006].

Doll, E. 1936. The Vineland School Maturity Scale. Publication of the training school at Vineland. *Dept. of Research Series*, 3: April.

Donnellan, E. 2004. Goodbye health boards, hello HSE, Health Supplement, *The Irish Times*. 28 December, Dublin: 1.

Donnelly-Cox, G. and O'Regan, A. 1998. *The Irish Voluntary Sector: A Case-Based Exploration of Organisational Growth Patterns and Organisational Dynamics*. 'The Contribution of the Third Sector to Social, Economic and Political Change' ISTR Third International Conference, Geneva, Switzerland: Université de Genève.

Donoghue, F. 1998. *The Politicisation of Disadvantage in the Republic of Ireland: The Role Played by the Third Sector*. ISTR Third International Conference, Geneva, Switzerland: Université de Genève.

Donoghue, F. 2002. Reflecting the Relationships. An Exploration of the Relationships between the former Eastern Health Board and Voluntary Organisations in the Eastern Region, Eastern Regional Health Authority: Dublin.

Donoghue, F. 2007. Foundations in Ireland. In *The Politics of Foundations: Comparative Perspectives from Europe and Beyond*, edited by H.K. Anheier, and S. Daly. London: Routledge.

Donovan, R. and Williams. A. 2007. Home as Therapeutic Landscape: Family Caregivers Providing Palliative Care at Home. In *Therapeutic Landscapes*, edited by A. Williams. Aldershot: Ashgate, 199–218.

Dorn, M. and Laws, G. 1994. Social Theory, body politics, and medical geography: extending Kearns's invitation, *The Professional Geographer* 46: 106–110.

Douglas, A. and Philpot, T. 1998. *Caring and Coping: A Guide to Social Services*. London: Routledge.

Drake, R.F. 1999. *Understanding Disability Policies*. London: Macmillan.

Drewett, A.Y. 1999. Social Rights and Disability: the language of 'rights' in the community care policies. *Disability and Society*, 14(1), 115–28.

Dyck, I. 1995. Hidden Geographies: The Changing Lifeworlds of Women with Disabilities. *Social Science and Medicine*, 40(3), 307–20.

Dyck, I. 1998. Women with Disabilities and Everyday Geographies: Home Space and the Contested Body. In *Putting Health into Place: Landscape, Identity and Well Being*, edited by R. Kearns and W. Gesler. New York: Syracuse University Press, 102–19.

Eldergill, A. no date. *Guardianship*, http://www.mentalhealthlawyers.com/Articles%20pdf%20web/Guardianship.pdf [accessed 17 February 2005].

Emerson, E. 2007. Poverty and people with intellectual disabilities. *Mental Retardation and Developmental Disabilities Research Reviews*. 13(2), 107–13.

Encylopedia of Philosophy. 2001. *John Locke, 1632–1704*. http://www.iep.utm.edu/l/locke.htm [accessed 23 August, 2004].

Enright, O. 2009. Quoted in 'Government scraps plan to publish carers' strategy', *The Irish Times*, Tuesday 3 March 2009.

Esping-Andersen, G. 1990. *The Three Worlds of Welfare Capitalism*. Cambridge: Polity Press.

Esping-Andersen, G. 1999. *Social Foundations of Postindustrial Economies*. Oxford: Oxford University Press.

Esping-Andersen, G. 2000. Three Worlds of Welfare Capitalism. In *The Welfare State Reader*, edited by C. Pierson, and F.G. Gastles. Cambridge: Polity Press, 154–69.

European Commission. 2009. *Report of the Ad Hoc Expert Group on the Transition from Institutional to Community-based Care*. European Commission.

Evans, D. 1983. *The Lives of Mentally Retarded People*. Boulder, CO: Westview Press.

Family Caregiver Alliance. 2003a. *About FCA*. http://www.caregiver.org/caregiver/jsp/content_node.jsp?nodeid=349 [accessed 10 October 2008].

Family Caregiver Alliance. 2003b. *Fact Sheet: New Medicare: What Caregivers Need to Know*. http://www.caregiver.org/caregiver/jsp/content_node.jsp?nodeid=890 [accessed 18 October 2008].

FÁS. 2010. Supported Employment Programme http://www.fas.ie/en/Communities/Supported+Employment.htm [accessed 29 February 2010].

Fast, J.E., Kolodinsky, J. and Hong, G.-S. 1998. The Hidden Costs of Informal Caregiving: An international comparison. *Consumer Interests Annual*, 44, 206–10.

Feinberg, L.F. and Pilisuk, T.L. 1999. *Survey of Fifteen States' Caregiver Support Programs: Final Report*. California: Family Caregiver Alliance.

Ferguson, P.M. 2004. The legacy of the almshouse. In *Mental Retardation in America,* edited by S. Noll, and J. Trent Jr. New York: New York University Press, 40–64.

Finch, J. 1989. *Family Obligations and Social Change*. Cambridge: Polity Press.

Finch, J. and Groves, D. 1983. *A Labour of Love: Women, Work and Caring*. London: Routledge.

Finch, J. and Mason, J. 1999. Obligations of Kinship in Contemporary Britain: Is there Normative Agreement? In *The Sociology of the Family: A Reader*, edited by G. Allan. Oxford: Blackwell.

Finnane, M. 1981. *Insanity and the Insane in Post-Famine Ireland*. London: Croom and Noble.

Fisher, I. 1998. Families Providing Complex Medical Care, Tubes and All. *The New York Times*. 7 June, New York, 1.

Fogerty, W. 1867. On the Planning of Lunatic Asylums. *The Irish Builder*, 9(172), 29–40.

Foucault, M. 1979. *Discipline and Punish: The Birth of the Prison*. New York: Vintage.

Foucault, M. 1982. *Madness and Civilisation: A History of Insanity in the Age of Reason*. London: Tavistock.

Foucault, M. 1986. *The Care of the Self*. R. Hurley (trans). Harmondsworth: Penguin.

Fox-Grage, W., Coleman, B. and Blancato, R.B. 2001. *Federal and State Policy in Family Caregiving: Recent Victories but Uncertain Future. Policy Brief No. 2*. Washington D.C: Family Caregiver Alliance.

Friedland, R.B. 1997. Financing Long-Term Care. In *Home-Based Care for a New Century*, edited by D.M. Fox and C. Raphael. Oxford: Blackwell Publishers and Millbank Memorial Fund.

Fyfe, N. and Milligan, C. 2003. Out of the shadows: exploring contemporary geographies of voluntarism, *Progress in Human Geography*, 27(4), 397–413.

Gastaldo, D. Andrews, G.J. and Khanlou, N. 2004. Therapeutic landscapes of the mind: theorizing some intersections between health geography, health promotion and immigration studies. *Critical Public Health*, 14(2), 157–76.
Gatrell, A.C. 2002. *Geographies of Health: An Introduction*. Oxford: Blackwell.
George, V. and Taylor-Gooby, P. (eds), 1996. *European Welfare Policy: Squaring the Welfare Circle*. London: Macmillan Press Ltd.
Geores, M. and Gesler, W.M. 1999. Compromised Space: Contests over the Provision of a Therapeutic Environment for People with Mental Illness. In *Therapeutic Landscapes: The Dynamic Between Place and Wellness*, edited by A. Williams. New York: Oxford University Press, 99–121.
Gesler, W.M. 1992. Therapeutic landscapes: medical issues in light of the new cultural geography. *Social Science and Medicine*, 34, 735–46.
Gibson-Graham, J.K. 1996. *The End of Capitalism as We Knew It: A Feminist Critique of Political Economy*. Oxford: Blackwell Publishers.
Gierke, O. 1990. *Political Theories of the Middle Age*. Cambridge: Cambridge University Press.
Gleeson, B. 1999. *Geographies of Disability*. London: Routledge.
Gleeson, B. and Kearns, R. 2001. Remoralising landscapes of care. *Environment and Planning D: Society and Space* 19, 61–80.
Glendinning, C. 2009. *Cash for care: implications for carers,* Geneva Association Health and Ageing Newsletter, 21, 3–6.
Glendinning, C., Arksey, H., Jones, K., Moran, N., Netten, A. and Rabiee, P. 2009. *Individual budgets: Impacts and outcomes for carers*. Research Findings, Social Policy Research Unit.
Goffman, E. 1961. *Asylums: Essays on the Social Situation of Mental Patients and Other Inmates*. New York: Doubleday.
Goodwin, S. 1997. *Community Care and the Future of Mental Health Welfare Provision*. Avebury: Aldershot.
Government of Ireland. 2006. *Towards 2016*. Dublin: Stationery Office.
Graham, H. 1999. The Informal Sector of Welfare: A crisis in caring? In *The Sociology of the Family*, edited by G. Allan. London: Blackwell.
Griffiths, Sir R. 1988. *Community Care: Agenda for Action*, London: HMSO.
Grogan, V. 1978. 'Towards the new constitution' in *The Years of the Great Test, 1926–39*, edited by F. MacManus. Dublin: Mercier Press.
Hall, E. 2000. 'Blood, brain and bones': taking the body seriously in the geography of health and impairment. *Area*, 32(1), 21–9.
Hall, E. and Kearns, R. 2001. Making space for the 'intellectual' in geographies of disability. *Health & Place*, 7(3), 237–45.
Hall, E. 2005. 'The entangled geographies of social exclusion/inclusion for people with learning disabilities', *Health & Place* 11(2), 107–15.
Hanly Report. 2003. Report of the National Task Force on Medical Staffing. *Hanly report*. Dublin: Stationery Office.
Hannigan, J.A. 1990. Containing the Luciferine spark: the Catholic Church and recent movements for social change in the Republic of Ireland. In *Sociological*

Studies in Roman Catholicism, edited by R. O'Toole. Leviston, NY: Edwin Mellen Press.
Harbert, W. and Rogers, P. (eds), 1983. *Community-based Social Care: The Avon Experience*. London: Bedford Square Press.
Harvey, D. 1982. *The Limits to Capital*. Oxford: Blackwell.
Haslanger, K. 2003. *Medicaid Managed Care in New York: A Work in Progress*. New York: United Hospital Fund.
Hatton, C., Robertson, J., Power, A., Baines, S. and Emerson, E. 2009. *Summary of Responses to the Consultation on Valuing People Now: From Progress to Transformation.* CeDR Research Report, London: HM Government.
Hawkesworth, M. 2001. Disabling Spatialities and the Regulation of a Visible Secret. *Urban Studies*, 38(2), 299–318.
Health & Place. 1997. Special Issue: Space, Place and the Asylum, *Health & Place*, 3(2), 71–141.
Health & Place. 2000. Special Issue: Post-Asylum Geographies, *Health & Place*, 6(2), 67–134.
Health & Place. 2005. Special Issue: Geographies of Intellectual Disability. *Health & Place,* 11(2), 77–195.
Heller, T.C. 1997. Modernity, Membership, and Multiculturalism. *Stanford Humanities Review*, 5(2).
Higgens, P. 1992. *Making Disability*. Springfield, IL: Charles Thomas.
Hills, J. 1998. *Thatcherism, New Labour and the Welfare State*. Centre for Analysis of Social Exclusion. CASE paper, CASE/13 August, London: London School of Economics.
HM Treasury. 1979. Balance of payments flows and monetary aggregates in the United Kingdom GES working paper No. 5, Treasury working paper No. 5. London: HMSO.
Holland, K. 2001. Older People would prefer care at home, says study. *The Irish Times*. 20 June 2001. Dublin.
Holloway, S.L. 1999. Reproducing motherhood. In *Geographies of New Femininities*, edited by N. Laurie, C. Dwyer, S. Holloway, and F. Smith. Harlow: Longman.
Home Office. 1991. *1991 United Kingdom Census*. London: Office for National Statistics.
Hubbard, P., Bartley, B., Fuller, D. and Kitchin, R.M. 2002 *Thinking Geographically: Space, Theory and Contemporary Human Geography*. London: Continuum.
Huber, E. and Stephens, J.D. 2001. Welfare state and production regimes in the era of retrenchment. In *The New Politics of the Welfare State*, edited by P. Pierson. Oxford: Oxford University Press, 107–45.
Hutton, W. 1995. *The State We're In*. London: Vintage.
Imrie, R. 1996. *Disability and the City: International Perspectives*. London: Paul Chapman Publishing.
Inclusion Ireland. 2009. *Inclusion Ireland newsletter*, Issue 44, December 2009.

Inglis, T. 1987. *Moral Monopoly: The Catholic Church in Modern Irish Society*. Dublin: Gill and Macmillan.

Isin, E. and Wood, P.K. 1999. *Citizenship and Identity*. London: Sage.

Jackson, A. 1935. The relation of hypothyroidism and mental deficiency. *Journal of Psycholo-asthenics* 40, 92–5.

Johnston, R.J. 1986. *Philosophy and Human Geography: An Introduction to Contemporary Approaches*. London: Edward Arnold Publishers.

Jones, D.W. 2002. *Myths, Madness, and the Family*. New York: Palgrave.

Joseph, A.E. and Phillips, D.R. 1984. *Accessibility and Utilization: Geographical Perspectives on Health Care Delivery*. New York: Harper & Row.

Kaiser Commission on Medicaid and the Uninsured. 2001. *Medicaid's Disabled Population and Managed Care*. March. Washington, D.C.: The Henry J. Kaiser Family Foundation.

Kaiser Commission on Medicaid and the Uninsured. 2002. *Medicaid Enrolment in the 50 States: A June 2002 Data Update*, June. Washington, D.C.: The Henry J. Kaiser Family Foundation.

Kaiser Commission on Medicaid and the Uninsured. 2003. *Bush Administration: Medicaid/SCHIP Proposal*. May. Washington, D.C.: The Henry J. Kaiser Family Foundation.

Kane, R. L. 1997. *Comparative National Policies on Care and Support of Older Persons*. 1997 World Congress of Gerontology, University of Minnesota, USA.

Kearney, N. and Skehill, C. 2005. *Social Work in Ireland: Historical Perspectives*. Dublin: Institute of Public Administration.

Kelly, F., Kelly, C., Maguire, G. and Craig S. 2009. *National Intellectual Disability Database Annual Report 2008*, HRB Statistics Series 6, HRB.

Keigher, S.M. and Stone, R. 1994. Payments for Care: The Case of the United States of America, in *Payments for Care*, edited by A. Evers, M. Pijl and C. Ungerson. Aldershot: Avebury, 321–45.

Kenny, K. 2004. *Ireland and the British Empire*. Oxford: Oxford University Press.

Kitchin, R. 1998. 'Out of place', 'knowing one's place': Towards a spatialised theory of disability and social exclusion. *Disability and Society*, 13(3), 343–56.

Kitchin, R. and Lysaght, K. 2003. Heterosexism and the geographies of everyday life in Belfast, Northern Ireland. *Environment and Planning A*, 35(3), 489–510.

Klass, G. 1985. 'Explaining America and the Welfare State: An Alternative Theory', *British J. of Political Science* 15, 427–50.

Klemm, J.D. 2000. Medicaid Spending: A Brief History. *Health Care Financing Review*, 22(1), 105–12.

KSAH. 2002. Chapter 13: Toward the 21st Century. http://www.americanhistory.or.kr/book/files/ethirteen01.html#132 [accessed 2 February 2008].

Land, H. and Rose, H. 1985. Compulsory Altruism for Some or an Altruistic Society for All? In *In Defence of Welfare*, edited by P. Bean, J. Ferris and D. Whynes. London: Tavistock.

Lane, P., McKenna, H.P., Ryan, A. and Fleming, P. 2000. *Listening to the voice of Carers: An Exploration of the Health and Social Care Needs and Experiences of Informal Carers of Older People*. Ireland: South Eastern Health Board.

Lash, S. and Urry J. 1987. *The End of Organized Capitalism*. London: Polity Press.

Laws, G. and Radford, J. 1998. Place, identity and disability: narratives of intellectually disabled people in Toronto. In *Putting Health into Place: Landscape, Identity and Well-being*, edited by R. Kearns and W. Gesler. Syracuse: Syracuse University Press.

Le Plante, M.P., Kennedy, J., Kaye, H.S. and Wenger, B.L. 1997. Disability and employment. *Disability Statistics Abstract*. No. 11, 30 January. California: Disability Statistics Center, University of California.

Leat, D. and Ungerson, C. 1994. Payments for Care: The Case of Great Britain, in *Payments for Care,* edited by A. Evers, M. Pijl and C. Ungerson. Aldershot: Avebury, Chapter 15.

Levine, C. and Zuckerman, C. 2000. Hands On/Hands Off: Why Health Care Professionals Depend on Families but Keep Them at Arm's Length. *The Journal of Law, Medicine, and Ethics*, 28(1), 5–18.

Levin-Epstein, M. 2000. How We Got It Anyway: The Clinton Health Plan Never Died. *Managed Care Magazine*, October.

Lewis, J. and Glennerster, H. 1996. *Implementing the New Community Care*. Milton Keynes Open University Press.

Lewis, J. 1999. The Concepts of Community Care and Primary Care in the UK: The 1960s to the 1990s. *Health and Social Care in the Community*, 7(5), 333–341

Lloyd, L. 2000. Caring about carers: only half the picture? *Critical Social Policy*, 20(1), 136–50.

Lonergan, E. 2000. *St Joseph's Hospital, Clonmel*. Published by author.

Luk, W.S.-C. 2002. The home care experience as perceived by the caregivers of Chinese dialysis patients. *International Journal of Nursing Studies*, 39(3), 269–77.

Macintyre, S., Maciver, S. and Sooman, A. 1993. Area, class and health; should we be focusing on people or places? *Journal of Social Policy*, 22, 213–34.

Mann, C. 2002. *The New Era of Medicaid Waivers*. September. Georgetown: University Institute for Health Care Research and Policy and Council on Health Care Economics and Policy.

Mansell, J. and Ericsson, K. 1996. *Deinstitutionalization and Community Living: Intellectual Disability Services in Britain, Scandinavia and the USA*. London: Chapman and Hall.

Manthorpe, J. 1994. The Family and Informal Care. In *Implementing Community Care,* edited by N. Malin. Buckingham: Open University Press.

Marmor, T., Mashaw, J. and Harvey, P. 1991. *America's Misunderstood Welfare State: Persistent Myths, Enduring Realities*. New York: Basic Books.

Marshall, T.H. 1950. *Citizenship and Social Class and Other Essays*. Cambridge: Cambridge University Press.

Marshall, T.H. 1977. Value Problems of Welfare-Capitalism, in *Welfare in Action*, edited by M. Fitzgerald, P. Halmos, J. Muncie and D. Zeldin. London and Henley: Routledge and Kegan Paul, in association with The Open University Press.

Marshall, T.H. 1981. *The Right to Welfare and Other Essays*. London: Heinemann.

Maryam, N.-W., Feldman, P.H., Gould, D.A., Levine, C., Kuerbis, A.N. and Donelan, K. 2002. When the Caregiver Needs Care: The Plight of Vulnerable Caregivers. *American Journal of Public Health*, 92(3), 409–13.

Mayer, D.N. 1994. Clinton Health Plan: The Wrong Prescription. *On Principle* 2,1.

McCarron, D. 1991 *Church power in the south...Home rule or Rome rule?*, http://flag.blackened.net/revolt/ws91/church32.html [accessed 1 October 2003].

McGrath, S. and Clutterbuck, P. 1998. *Third Sector Transformation in an Emerging City State: A Case Study of the Toronto Social Planning Council*. Université de Genéve, Geneva, Switzerland: ISTR Third International Conference.

McLaughlin, E. 1993. Ireland: Catholic Corporatism. In *Comparing Welfare States: Britain in International Context*, edited by A. Cochrane, and J. Clarke. London: Sage, in association with the Open University, 205–37.

McMahon, M. and Barron, B. 2004. *EUROFAMCARE: National Background Report for Ireland*. Hamburg, Germany: European Union.

Meade, M.S. and Earickson, R.J. 2000. *Medical Geography*. London: Guilford Press.

Merriman, B. and Canavan, J. 2007. *Towards best practice in the provision of respite services for people with intellectual disabilities and autism*. NUI Galway: Child and Family Research Centre.

Metzel, D.S. 2004. Historical Social Geography. In *Mental Retardation in America*, edited by S. Noll, and J. Trent Jr. New York: New York University Press, 420–44.

Midland Health Board. 2004. *Dementia Working Group Progress Report*. February 2004.

Milligan, C. 2000. Bearing the burden: towards a restructured geography of caring. *Area*, 32(1), 49–58.

Milligan, C. 2001. *Geographies of Care: space, place and the voluntary sector*. Aldershot, Ashgate.

Milligan, C. 2009. *There's No Place like Home: People, Place and Care in an Ageing Society*. Aldershot: Ashgate.

Milligan, C. and Conradson, D. (eds), 2006. *Geographies of Voluntarism: New Spaces of Health, Welfare and Governance*. Bristol: Policy Press.

Milligan, C. and Fyfe, N. 2004. Putting the voluntary sector in its place: geographical perspectives on voluntarism and social welfare, *Journal of Social Policy*, 33(1), 73–93.

Milligan, C. and Power, A. 2009. The Changing Geography of Care. In *Companion to Human Geography*, edited by T. Brown, S. McLafferty and G. Moon. London: Blackwell.

Milne, D., Pitt, I. and Sabin, N. 1993. Evaluation of a carer support scheme for elderly people: the importance of 'coping', *British Journal of Social Work*, 23(2), 157–68.

Moriarty, J. and Webb, S. 2000. *Part of their Lives: Community Care for Older People with Dementia*. Bristol: The Policy Press.

Morris, J. 1991. *Pride Against Prejudice*. London: Women's Press.

Morris, J. 1993. *Independent Lives? Community Care and Disabled People*. Basingstoke: Macmillan.

Mouffe, C. 1996. Radical Democracy or Liberal Democracy. In *Radical Democracy: Identity, Citizenship, and the State*, edited by D. Trend. London: Routledge.

Mouffe, C. 2005. *The Return of the Political*. London: Verso.

Muckross Research Library. no date. *Ireland in the 1930s–1940s*, http://www.muckross-house.ie/library_files/ireland_in_the_30s.htm [accessed 7 April 2005].

Murphy, N., Christian, B., Caplin, D. and Young, P. 2007. The health of caregivers for children with disabilities: caregiver perspectives. *Child Care Health Development*, 33(2), 180–7.

Murray, I. 1994. Supported Employment Programme. *Working Brief* 55. June, 45–98.

NAMHI 2003. Newsletter, August http://www.namhi.ie [accessed 25 April 2007].

NAMHI 2004. Homepage, http://www.namhi.ie/namfr/namfnl.htm [accessed 23 February 2007].

National Archives of Ireland. 2004. *Research guide to the records of the Poor Law*. http://www.nationalarchives.ie/research/poor_law.htm [accessed 30 March 2005].

National Association of State Budget Officers (NASBO). 2009. *2008 State Expenditure Report*. Washington D.C.: NASBO.

National Council for the Elderly. 1994. *Support Services for Carers of Elderly People Living at Home*. Dublin: National Council for the Elderly.

National Disability Authority. 2004. *Towards Best Practice in Provision of Health Services for People with Disabilities in Ireland*. Dublin: NDA.

National Economic and Social Council. 1987. *Community Care Services: An overview*. Report 84, Sheila O'Connor. Dublin: National Economic and Social Council.

National Family Caregivers Association. 2000. *54 Million Americans Involved in Family Caregiving Last Year*, http://www.nfcacares.org.[accessed 14 March 2002].

National Primary Care Research and Development Centre. 2005. *Equity in the distribution of primary care in relation to population need: the generality of inverse care*, http://www.npcrdc.man.ac.uk/ResearchDetail.cfm?ID=14 [accessed 1 April 2005].

National Sound Archive. 2000. *Family Life and Work Experience Before 1918*. British Library, London.

Nehring, W.M. 2004. Formal health care at the community level. In *Mental Retardation in America*, edited by S. Noll, and J. Trent Jr. New York: New York University Press, 371–83.
Nerney, T. no date. *The Purpose of Public Funding for Individuals with Disabilities*. Michigan: Centre for Self-Determination.
Newcomer, R.J., Fox, P.J. and Harrington, C.A. 2001. Health and long-term care for people with Alzheimer's disease and related dementias: policy research issues. *Aging and Mental Health* 5. Supplement 1, 124–37.
NHS 2005. Stratetgic Health Authorities, http://www.NHS.co.uk [accessed 13 April 2005].
NHS 2010. The NHS Confederation, http://www.nhsconfed.org/Pages/home.aspx [accessed 22 March 2010].
Neufeld, A., Harrison, M.J., Hughes, K. and Stewart, M. 2007. Non-supportive interactions in the experience of women family caregivers. *Health and Social Care in the Community*, 15(6), 530–41.
Nirje, B. 1969. The normalization principle and its human management implications, in *Changing Patterns in Residential Services for the Mentally Retarded*, edited by R. Kugel and W. Wolfensberger. Washington, D.C.: President's Committee on Mental Retardation.
Nolan, K.A., Trahar, M.F., Clarke, C. and Blass, J.P. 1993. Respite-retreat for dementia caregivers: A demonstration, *American Journal of Alzheimer's Disease and Other Dementias*, 8(1), 34–8.
Noll, S. and Trent, J.W. 2004. *Mental Retardation in America: A Historical Reader*. New York: New York University Press.
Nugent, J. 1858. *Observations on the Report of the Commissioners of Inquiry into Lunatic Asylums and other Institutions for the Custody and Treatment of the Insane in Ireland, in a Letter to the Right Honourable Lord Viscount Naas, M.P. Chief Secretary*. J. Nugent M.D., Inspector of Lunatic Asylums, Her Majesty's Stationery Office.
Oberlander, J. 2003. *The Politics of Medicare Reform*. IHHCPAR Seminar, 16 October, Rutgers University: Institute for Health, Health Care Policy and Aging Research.
O'Brien, M. and Penna, S. 1998. *Theorising Welfare: Enlightenment and Modern Society*. London: Sage Publications.
O'Connell, M. 2000. Can Blessed Martin still shine with Health?, *The Sunday Business Post*. 30 January, Dublin.
O'Donovan, O. 1997. Contesting Concepts of Care: The Case of the Home Help Service in Ireland. In *The Sociology of Health and Illness in Ireland*, edited by A. Cleary and M. Treacy. London: Blackwell Publishers, 140–53.
Oliver, M. 1983. *Social Work and Disabled People*. Basingstoke: Macmillan.
Oliver, M. 1990. *The Politics of Disablement*. London: Routledge.
Oliver, M. 1996. *Understanding Disability: From Theory to Practice*. Basingstoke: Macmillan.

Oliver, M. and Barnes, C. 1998. *Disabled People and Social Policy: From Exclusion to Inclusion.* London: Longman.

O'Louglin, A. 2005. Social Policy and Older People. In *Contemporary Irish Social Policy*, edited by S. Quin, P. Kennedy, A. O'Donnell, and G. Kiely. Dublin: University College Dublin Press.

Opie, A. Fulcher, L Hawke, G. and Allen, N. 1992. *There's Nobody There: Community Care of Confused Older People.* Philadelphia, PA: University of Pennsylvania Press.

O'Shaughnessy, C., Lyke, B. and Storey, J.R. 2002. *CRS Report for Congress: Long-Term Care: What Direction for Public Policy?* The Library of Congress, Washington D.C.: Congressional Research Service.

Our Healthier Nation. 2004. *Primary Care Groups*, http://www.ohn.gov.uk/ohn/partnerships/primary.htm [accessed 22 February 2005].

Pakulski, J. 1997. Cultural Citizenship. *Citizenship Studies*, 1: 73–86.

Parr, H. 1997. Mental health, public space, and the city: questions of individual and collective access. *Environment and Planning D: Society and Space*, 15, 435–54.

Parr, H. 2002. Medical Geography: diagnosing the body in medical and health geography, 1999–2000. *Progress in Human Geography*, 26 (2), 240–51.

Paton, C. 1999. New Labour's health policy: the new healthcare state, in *New Labour, New Welfare State?* edited by M. Powell. Bristol: Policy Press.

Peillon, M. 2001. *Welfare in Ireland: Actors, Resources and Strategies*. London: Praeger.

Percy, S.L. 2001. Disability Policy in the United States: Policy, in *Disability and Federalism: Comparing Different Approaches to Full Participation*, edited by D. Cameron, and V. Fraser. London: McGill-Queens University Press, 231–68.

Petersen, A. and Lupton, P. 1996. *The New Public Health: Health and Self in the Age of Risk.* London: Sage.

Pfaller, A., Gough, I. and Therborn, G. 1991. The issue. In *Can the Welfare State Compete?* edited by A. Pfaller, I. Gough and G. Therborn. London: Macmillan.

Pfeiffer, D. 2001. The Changing Nature of Disability Policy and its Distributive Impact. *Disability Studies Quarterly*, 21(4), 158–76.

Phillips, B., Mahoney, K., Simon-Rusinowitz, L., Schore, J., Barrett, S., Ditto, W., Reimers, T. and Doty, P. 2003. *Lessons from the Implementation of Cash and Counseling in Arkansas, Florida, and New Jersey*. June. New Jersey: The Robert Wood Johnson Foundation, U.S. Department of Health and Human Services, Office of The Assistant Secretary for Planning and Evaluation.

Phillips, J. 2009. *Care: Key Concepts.* London: Polity Press.

Philo, C. 1987. 'Fit localities for an asylum': the historical geography of the 'mad business' in England viewed through the pages of the Asylum Journal. *Journal of Historical Geography*, 13, 398–415.

Pickard, L. 2001. Carer Break or Carer-blind? Policies for Informal Carers in the UK. *Social Policy and Administration*, 35 (4), 441–58.

Pinch, S. 1985. *Cities and Services: The Geography of Collective Consumption*. London: Routledge.
Pinch, S. 1997. *Worlds of Welfare: Understanding the Changing Geographies of Social Welfare Provision*. London: Routledge.
Pinfold, V. 2000. 'Building up safe havens…all around the world': users' experiences of living in the community with mental health problems. *Health & Place*, 6(3), 201–12.
Plowden, W. 2003. The Compact: Attempts to Regulate Relationships between Government and the Voluntary Sector in England, Nonprofit and Voluntary. *Voluntary Sector Quarterly*, 32(3).
Polivka, L. 2001. *Paying Family Members to Provide Care: Policy Considerations for States: Policy Brief No. 7*. Washington, D.C.: Family Caregiver Alliance.
Porter, R. 1992. Madness and its institutions. In *Medicine in Society: Historical Essays*, edited by A. Wear. Cambridge: Cambridge University Press, 277–302.
Powell, F. 1998. The Professional Challenges of Reflexive Modernization: Social Work in Ireland. *British Journal of Social Work* 28, 311–28.
Powell, F. and Guerin, D. 1997. *Civil Society and Social Policy*. Dublin: A. and A. Farmar.
Powell, J.L. 2001. The NHS and Community Care Act 1990. In *The United Kingdom: A Critical Review*, http://sincronia.cucsh.udg.mx/nhs.htm [accessed 12 August 2003].
Powell, M. and Boyne, G. 2001. The Spatial Strategy of Equality and the Spatial Division of Welfare. *Social Policy and Administration*, 35(2), 181–95.
Power, A. and Kenny, A. When Care's Left to Roam: Carers Experiences of Grassroots Nonprofit Services in Ireland. *Health & Place*. (forthcoming).
Prince, M.J. 2009. *Absent Citizens: Disability Politics and Policy in Canada*. Ontario: University of Toronto Press.
Prior, P.M. 2003. Dangerous lunacy: The misuse of mental health law in nineteenth-century Ireland. *Journal of Forensic Psychiatry and Psychology* 14(3), 525–41.
Programme for Economic and Social Progress. 1991. *Report of Programme for Economic and Social Progress*. Dublin: Stationery Office.
Prospectus and Watson Wyatt. 2003. Audit of the structure and functions of the Irish healthcare system (known as the Prospectus Report). Dublin: Department of Health.
Quin, S. 2005. Improving Health Care: Health Policy in Ireland, in *Contemporary Irish Social Policy*, edited by S. Quin, P. Kennedy, A. O'Donnell and K. Gabriel. Dublin: University College Dublin Press.
Quin, S., Kennedy, P., O'Donnell, A. and Gabriel, K. 2005. *Contemporary Irish Social Policy*. Dublin: University College Dublin Press.
Quin, S. and Redmond, B. 2005. Moving from Needs to Rights: Social Policy for People with Disability in Ireland. In *Contemporary Irish Social Policy,* edited by S. Quin, P. Kennedy, A. O'Donnell and K. Gabriel. Dublin: University College Dublin Press.

Radford, J. and Phillips, D. 1985. Closure of major institutions for the mentally handicapped: geographical evidence from a case study in Southwest England. *South West Papers in Geography*, Occasional Series, 10.

Ramon, S. 1991. *Beyond Community Care*. London: Macmillan Education Ltd.

Ramsay, D. 1958. *Report of a special inspection of Clonmel District Mental Hospital*, Assistant Inspector for Mental Hospitals.

Redden, C.J. 2002. *Health Care, Entitlement, and Citizenship*. Toronto, University of Toronto Press.

Redmond, B. 1996. *Listening to Parents: the aspirations, expectations and anxieties of parents about their teenager with learning disability*. Family Studies Centre, University College Dublin.

Reinhard, S. 2001. *The Work of Caregiving: What do ADLs and IADLs Tell Us?* Presented at ADL-IADL Working Group Meeting: 'Toward a New Job Description for Family Caregivers: Moving Beyond ADLs-IADLs', United Hospital Fund, New York.

Report of The Mental Deficiency Committee (Wood Report). 1929. London: HMSO.

Richards, P.L. 2004. 'Beside her sat her idiot child', in S. Noll and W. Trent Jr. *Mental Retardation in America*. New York: New York University Press, 65–87.

Richardson, S. 1996. The role of women in electoral politics in Yorkshire during the eighteen-thirties', *Northern History* 19.

Riley, T. 2002. *State Health Policy Responses to Recessions, 1970–2002. What have we learned? Where are we headed?* Portland, ME: National Academy for State Health Policy.

Rimmer, L. 1983. The economics of work and caring. In *A Labour of Love: Women, Work, and Caring*, edited by J. Finch and D. Groves. London: Routledge and Kegan Paul.

Ritzer, G. and Goodman, D.J. 2003. *Sociological Theory*. New York: McGraw Hill.

RNID. 1999. *Social Security Committee Inquiry: The contributory principle*, www.rnid.org.uk/docs/welfare_benefits/ contributory_principle.doc [accessed 18 November 2004].

Roberts, A. 2001. *The Lunacy Commission, A Study of Its Origin, Emergence and Character: Mental History Timeline*, http://www.mdx.ac.uk/www/study/mhhtim.htm [accessed 18 November 2004].

Robins, J. 1986. *Fools and Mad: A History of the Insane in Ireland*. Dublin: Institute of Public Administration.

Robinson, C. and Williams, V. 2002. Carers of People with Learning Disabilities and their Experiences of the 1995 Carers Act. *British Journal of Social Work*. 32(2) 169–83.

Rogers, A. and Pilgrim, D. 2001. *Mental Health Policy in Britain. 2nd Edition.* Basingstoke: Palgrave Macmillan.

Rolph, S. and Walmsley, J. 2006. Oral History and New Orthodoxies: Narrative Accounts in the History of Learning Disability, *Oral History*, Spring, 81–91.

Rose, G. 1993. *Feminism and Geography: The Limits of Geographical Knowledge*. Cambridge: Polity Press.
Rosenbaum, S. 2001. *Olmstead v L.C.: Implications for Family Caregivers. Policy Brief No. 6*. Washington, D.C.: Family Caregiver Alliance.
Rosenberg, H. 1987. Motherwork, stress and depression: The costs of privatized social reproduction. In *Feminism and the Political Economy: Women's Work, Women's Struggles*, edited by H.J. Maroney and M. Luxton. Toronto: Methuen, 181–96.
Royal Commission. 1957. *Report of the Royal Commission on the Law Relating to Mental Illness and Mental Deficiency,* London: HMSO.
Ruddle, H. 1994. *Caring for the Carers: Guidelines for Good Practice*. Republic of Ireland: Soroptimist International
Ruggie, M. 1996. *Realignments in the Welfare State: health policy in the United States, Britain, and Canada*. New York: Columbia University Press.
Rummery, K., Ellis, K. and Davis, A. 1999. Negotiating Access to Assessments: Perspectives of front-line workers, people with disabilities and carers. *Health and Social Care in the Community*, 7(4), 296–300.
Rummery, K. and Glendinning, C. 2000. Access to Services as a Civil and social Rights Issue: The Role of Welfare professionals in Regulating Access to and commissioning Services for Disabled and Older People under New Labour. *Social Policy and Administration*, 34(5), 529–50.
Ryan, A. 1999. *Walls of Silence*. Kilkenny: Red Lion Press.
Ryan, J. and Thomas, F. 1987. *The Politics of Mental Handicap*. London: Free Association Books.
Ryan, S. 2008. 'I used to worry about what other people thought but now I just think…well I don't care': shifting accounts of learning difficulties in public places, *Health & Place*, 23(3), 199–210.
Salamon, L.M., Sokolowski, S.W. and List, R. 2003. *Global Civil Society: An Overview*. Baltimore, MD: The Johns Hopkins Center for Civil Society Studies.
Salazar, C. 2003. Demographic Growth and the 'Cultural Factor' in Ireland: rethinking the relationship between structure and event. *History and Anthropology*, 14(3), 271–81.
Schultz, S.K. 2004. *The Dawn of Liberalism: Progressivism*, http://us.history.wisc.edu/hist102/lectures/lecture11.html [accessed 15 April 2005].
Scorfield, M. 1999. *Establishing and forming partnerships between voluntary organisations and the statutory sector in the current political and economic climate: learning from past mistakes*, www.socialworksearch.com/research/researchms2.shtml [accessed 22 May 2002].
Scull, A. 1993. *The Most Solitary of Afflictions: Madness and Society in Britain 1700–1900*. New Haven and London: Yale University Press.
Seddon, D., Robinson, C., Reeves, C., Tommis, T., Woods, B. and Russell, I. 2007. In their Own Right: Translating the Policy of Carer Assessment into Practice, *British Journal of Social Work*, 37(8), 1335–52.

Seebohm Report. 1968. *Report of the Committee on Local Authority and Allied Personal Social Services*, Cmnd, 2702, London: HMSO.

Shakespeare, T. 2000. *The Disability Reader*, London: Continuum.

Sibley, D. 1995. *Geographies of Exclusion: Society and Difference in the West*. London: Routledge.

Sibley, D. 2001. The Binary City. *Urban Studies,* 38(2), 239–50.

Signposts. 2003. *Annual Report 1st April 2002 to 31st March 2003*. Morecambe: Signposts Reg. Charity.

Silberberg, M. 2001. *Respite Care: State Policy Trends and Model Programs. Policy Brief No. 4*. Washington D.C.: Family Caregiver Alliance.

Simons, K. and Watson, D. 1999. *The View From Arthur's Seat. A literature review of housing and support options 'beyond Scotland'*, http://www.scotland.gov.uk/cru/kd01/view-07.htm [accessed 25 February 2005].

Skinner, D., Slattery, E. and Lachicotte, W. 2002. *Disability, Health Coverage, and Welfare Reform*, October. Washington D.C.: The Henry J. Kaiser Foundation.

Smith, A. 1776. *An Inquiry into the Nature and Causes of the Wealth of Nations*, http://www.adamsmith.org/smith/won-index.htm [accessed 25 March, 2004].

Smith, G., O'Keeffe, J., Carpenter, L., Doty, P., Kennedy, G., Burwell, B., Mollica, R. and Williams, L. 2000. *Understanding Medicaid Home and Community Services: A Primer*, October. Washington, D.C.: U.S. Department of Health and Human Services, Office of the Assistant Secretary for Planning and Evaluation.

Smith, M. 2006. *Mental Retardation and Developmental Delay: Genetic and Epigenetic Factors*. New York: Oxford University Press.

Smith, V., Gifford, K., Ramesh, R. and Wachino, V. 2003. *Medicaid Spending Growth: A 50–State Update for Fiscal Year 2003*, January. Washington, D.C.: The Kaiser Commission on Medicaid and the Uninsured.

Social Security Online. 2003. *The History of Social Security*, http://www.ssa.gov/history/history.html [accessed 15 October 2006].

Soja, E. 1996. *Thirdspace*. London: Blackwell.

Soldo, B.J. and Freedman, V.A. 1994. Care of the Elderly: Division of Labour Among the Family, Market, and State. In *Demography of Aging*, edited by L. G. Martin and S.H. Preston. Open Book, The National Academy of Sciences.

Spicker, P. 2003. *An Introduction to Social Policy*, http://www2.rgu.ac.uk/publicpolicy/ [accessed 9 September 2006].

Stone, M. 1985. Shellshock and the psychologists. In W.F. Bynum, R.Porter and M. Shepherd (eds), *The Anatomy of Madness. Vol 2*. London: Tavistock.

Stone, R. 1999. *Long-Term Care: Coming of Age in the 21st Century*. Wisconsin: Family Impact Seminars, The Policy Institute for Family Impact Seminars.

Stone, R. 2001. Providing Long-Term Care Benefits in Cash: moving to a disability model. *Health Affairs*, 20(6), 96–108.

Spencer, H. 1857. Progess: Its Law and Causes, *The Westminster Review*, 67 (April), 445–65.

Swain, J., French, S. and Cameron, C. 2003. *Controversial Issues in a Disabling Society*. Buckingham, Open University Press.

Sweeney, P. 2004. If we want hospitals, then we will have to end the tax breaks, *The Irish Times*. 17 April, Dublin: 13.

Tanenbaum, S.J., and Hurley, R.E. 1995. Disability and the managed care frenzy: A cautionary note. *Health Affairs*, 14, 213–19.

Taylor, M. 1992. The Changing role of the Nonprofit Sector in Britain: Moving Towards the Market, in *Government and Third Sector*, edited by B. Gidron, et al. San Francisco: Jossey-Bass Publications.

The Irish Times. 2009. Government Scraps Plan to Publish Carer's Strategy. Breaking News, 3 March 2009.

Thomas, C. 2003. Developing the social relational in the social model of disability: a theoretical agenda, in *The Social Model of Disability – Theory and Research*, edited by C. Barnes. Leeds: The Disability Press.

Thomas, C. 2007. *Sociologies of Disability and Illness. Contested Ideas in Disability Studies and Medical Sociology*. Basingstoke: Palgrave Macmillan.

Thomas, C., and Morris, S.M. 2002. Informal Carers in Cancer Contexts. European *Journal of Cancer Care*, 11(3), 178–82.

Thomson, M. 1996. Family, Community, and State: The Micro-Politics of Mental Deficiency. In *From Idiocy to Mental Deficiency*, edited by J. Digby and D. Wright. London: Routledge, 207–30.

Thomson, R. G. 1997. *Extraordinary Bodies: Figuring Physical Disability in American Culture and Literature*. New York: Columbia University Press.

Titmuss, R. 1974. *Social Policy: An Introduction*. London: Allen and Unwin.

Tizard, J. 1960. Residential Care of Mentally Handicapped Children. *British Medical Journal*, 1041–46.

Tizard, J. 1964. *Community Services for the Mentally Handicapped*. London: Oxford University Press.

Torrey, E. and Miller, J. 2007. *The Invisible Plague: The Rise of Mental Illness from 1750 to the Present*. New Jersey: Rutgers University Press.

Townsend, P. 1995. The Structural Causes of Social Polarisation and Growing International Poverty. In *Global and Local: New York/London Through the Prism of Race, Class and Ethnicity*, edited by R. Franklin. Papers updated from a Conference organised by the Michael Harrington Center for Democratic Values and Social Change, April 30 – May 1, 1993. Minnesota: Minnesota University Press.

Townsend, P. 1957. *The Family Life of Old People*. London: Routledge and Kegan Paul.

Townsend, P. and Wedderburn, D. 1965. The aged in the Welfare State: the interim report of a survey of persons aged 65 and over in Britain, 1962 and 1963. London: Occasional Papers on Social Administration, No. 14.

Tufts Managed Care Institute. 1998. *A Brief History of Managed Care*, http://www.tmci.org/downloads/BriefHist.pdf [accessed 22 January 2008].

Twigg, J. 1992. Carers in the service system, in *Carers: Research and Practice*, edited by J. Twigg. London: HMSO.

Twigg, J. 2000. Carework as bodywork. *Ageing and Society*, 20, 389–411.

Twigg, J. and Atkin, K. 1994. *Carers Perceived: Policy and Practice in Informal Care*. Buckingham: Open University Press.

UK Government.1999. *Caring About Carers: A National Strategy for Carers*. London: HMSO.

UK Parliament. 1991. *Publications*, http://www.publications.parliament.uk/pa/cm199091/cmhansrd/1991–05–03/Writtens-2.html [accessed 17 January 2005].

UK Parliament. 1996. *House of Commons Hansard Debates for 18 Dec 1996*, http://www.parliament.the-stationery-office.co.uk/pa/cm199697/cmhansrd/vo961218/debtext/61218–41.htm [accessed 21 February 2005].

Ungerson, C. 1990. *Gender and Caring: Work and Welfare in Britain and Scandinavia*. London: Harvester Wheatsheaf.

Ungerson, C. 1995. Gender, cash and informal care; European perspectives and dilemmas. *Journal of Social Policy*, 24(1), 31–52.

Van Til, J. 2007. Wonderland 2006: The Nonprofit sector in the US. In *Differing Images: The Irish Nonprofit Sector and Comparative Perspectives*, edited by G. Donnelly-Cox and C. Breathnach. Dublin: The Liffey Press, 29–39.

Valentine, G. 2001. *Social Geographies: Space and Society*. London: Prentice Hall.

Walmsley, J. 2001. Normalisation, Emancipatory Research and Learning Disability, *Disability and Society*, 16(2), 187–205.

Walmsley, J. and Rolph, S. 2001. The Development of Community Care for People with Learning Difficulties 1913 to 1946. *Critical Social Policy*, 21(1), 59–80.

Walsh, T. 1999. Changing expectations: the impact of child 'protection' on Irish social work. *Child and Family Social Work* 4(1), 33–44.

Walsh, D. and Daly, A. 2004. *Mental illness in Ireland 1750–2002. Reflections on the Rise and Fall of Institutional Care*. Dublin: Health Research Board.

Warren, M. 2003. *A Chronology of State Medicine, Public Health, Welfare and Related Services in Britain: 1066–1999*, http://www.chronology.ndo.co.uk/index.htm [accessed 6 April 2005].

Watson, N., McKie, L., Hughes, B., Hopkins, D. and Gregory, S. 2004. Interdependence, Needs and Care: The Potential for Disability and Feminist Theorists to Develop an Emancipatory Model. *Sociology*, 38(2), 331–50.

Wearing, M. 1998. *Working in Community Services*. NSW, Australia: Allen and Unwin.

Webb, A. and Wistow, G. 1986. *Planning, Need and Scarcity: Essays on the Personal Social Services*. London: Allen and Unwin.

Webster, C. 2003. *Eugenic Sterilisation: Europe's Shame*, http://www.healthmatters.org.uk/stories/webster31.html [accessed 18 November, 2004].

Welfare.ie, 2004. Allowances and Benefits. http://www.welfare.ie [accessed 17 November 2004].

Welshman, J. and Walmsley, J. (eds), 2006. *Community Care in Perspective: Care, Control, and Citizenship*. Basingstoke: Palgrave.

Whitehouse. 2001. *National Family Caregivers Month, 2001*, http://www.whitehouse.gov/news/releases/2001/11/20011109–25.html [accessed 12 March 2002].

Wiles, J. 2003. Daily Geographies of Caregivers: mobility, routine, scale. *Social Science and Medicine*, 57, 1307–25.

Williams, A. 1996. The Development of Ontario's Home Care Program: A Critical Geographical Analysis. *Social Science and Medicine*, 42(6), 937–48.

Williams, A. 2002. Changing geographies of care: employing the concept of therapeutic landscapes as a framework in examining home space. *Social Science and Medicine*, 55(6), 141–54.

Williams, A. 2004. Shaping the Practice of Home Care: Critical Case Studies of the Significance of the Meaning of Home. *International Journal of Palliative Nursing*, 10(7), 333–42.

Williams, A. 1996. The Development of Ontario's Home Care Program: A Critical Geographical Analysis. *Social Science and Medicine*, 42(6), 937–48.

Wilson, J. 1982. *The Politics of Regulation*. London: Basic Books.

Wilson, K. 2003. Therapeutic Landscapes and First Nations Peoples: an exploration of culture, health and place, *Health & Place*, 9, 83–92.

Wilton, R., Dear, M., Gaber, S. J. and Takahashi, L. 1997. Seeing people differently: the sociospatial construction of disability. *Environment and Planning D: Society and Space*, 15, 455–80.

Wilton, R. 1998. The Constitution of Difference: Space and Psyche in Landscapes of Exclusion. *Geoforum*, 29(2), 173–85.

Winchester, M. and Frydman, D. 2003. *Financing Long-Term Care For People with Disabilities: Issue 2*. Spring, Franklin Pierce Law Center: The Policy Resource Center, Institute for Health, Law, and Ethics.

Wolch, J. and Philo, C. 2000. From distributions of deviance to definitions of difference: past and future mental health geographies. *Health & Place*, 6, 137–57.

Wolpert, J. 1976. Opening closed spaces. *Annals of the Association of American Geographers,* 66, 1–13.

Wolfenden Committee. 1978. *The Future of Voluntary Organisations.* London: HMSO.

World Health Organisation. 1961. *Statistics Report*, 14: 221–45. Geneva: World Health Organisation.

Wright, D. 2004. Mongols in our midst. In *Mental Retardation in America*, edited by S. Noll, and J. Trent Jr. New York: New York University Press, 92–119.

Wunderlich, G.S. and Kohler, P.O. 2001. *Improving the Quality of Long-Term Care*. Washington, D.C.: National Academy Press.

Wykle, M.L. 1994. Physical and mental health of women caregivers of older adults. *Journal of Gerontological Nursing*, 20(3), 48–9.

Index